Handbook on

HUMAN RESOURCES MANAGEMENT

for Healthcare Professionals

EUCHARIA E. NNADI

R.PH., J.D., PH.D.

HOWARD UNIVERSITY PRESS
Washington, D.C.
1997

Howard University Press, Washington, D.C. 20017

Manufactured in the United States of America

This book is printed on acid-free paper.

10 9 8 7 6 5 4 3 2 1

Library of Congress Cataloging-in-Publication Data

Nnadi-Okolo, Eucharia E., 1954–
    Handbook on human resources management for health care
professionals / Eucharia E. Nnadi-Okolo.
        p.   cm.
    ISBN 0-88258-195-3 (pbk.)
    1. Health facilities—Personnel management.   I. Title.
RA971.35.N65   1997
362.1′068′3—dc21   96-44092
                                                                            CIP

DEDICATION

To my mother,
Sister Lucy Anyamanwa Oguanobi-Nnadi,
who gave me the opportunity to receive a good
education, and encouraged me to reach
out for the best and to make each day
an improvement on the day before.

EUCHARIA E. NNADI, R.PH., J.D., PH.D.

Contents

List of Figures

Acknowledgments

I am most grateful to a large number of people who provided consultation, suggestions, technical help, and encouragement for this handbook. To Sheila Adiele, Evarista C. Nnadi, M.D., and Bridget Akazie for their support. To Leslie Washington and Iris Mitchell for their technical assistance. To Emmanuel N. Odimgbe, M.E.; Patricia Dike Odimgbe, M.D.; Jan McReynolds, Ph.D.; Arcelia Johnson-Fannin, Pharm.D.; and my mother, who has always encouraged and motivated me. I am grateful to my invaluable teachers: Albert I. Wertheimer, Ph.D.; Hugh Kabat, Ph.D.; William Tindall, Ph.D.; Johnnie E. Early, Ph.D.; Francis Schneider, Pharm.D.; and many others. I am also grateful to all those who buy this handbook; I hope that they find it useful.

EUCHARIA E. NNADI, R.PH., J.D., PH.D.

Preface

I hope that this handbook will provide a practical application of concepts and issues in human resources management for healthcare professionals. Too many healthcare professionals enter private practice and supervisory roles with very little knowledge of human resources management—an area that is vital not only for their practice to survive, but for successful overall management. Although some schools for health professionals now include a basic management course in their curriculum, such courses provide only a brief overview. Human resources textbooks specifically for health professionals are very limited and often do not include many of the issues addressed in this book. This book should help fill the void.

This handbook is designed for (1) healthcare professionals such as pharmacists, nurses, dentists, physicians, public health workers, optometrists, chiropractors, allied health professionals, and health policy makers who deal with personnel issues, either as a supervisor in an institutional setting (such as a hospital, nursing home, or administrative office) or as an owner or manager in private community-based practice; (2) students in any of the health professions who are contemplating entrepreneurship or a supervisory role in a healthcare setting, or in a healthcare policy or administrative setting; (3) healthcare professors teaching human resources management to students.

The handbook includes samples and guides, and covers important personnel issues such as conflict resolution, employee frustration, job burnout and stress management, employee pilferage, Total Quality Management (TQM), and legal and regulatory aspects of personnel management—workers' compensation, employment discrimination, the Age Discrimination in Employment Act, the Americans with Disabilities Act, the Family Medical Leave Act, the National Labor Relations Act, alternative dispute resolution (mediation and arbitration), and sexual harassment.

This handbook will, I hope, help healthcare practitioners, policy makers, professors, and students deal with human resources management issues and problems.

EUCHARIA E. NNADI, R.PH., J.D., PH.D.
Princess Anne, MD
1997

The Author

Eucharia E. Nnadi, R.Ph., J.D., Ph.D. is the Vice President of Academic Affairs at University of Maryland Eastern Shore. Prior to that she was the dean of the College of Pharmacy and Pharmaceutical Sciences at Howard University, Washington, D.C. She began her academic career as an assistant professor of pharmacy administration at the College of Pharmacy and Pharmaceutical Sciences, Florida A&M University (FAMU), in 1981 and became the first female tenured full professor at the college in 1989.

Dr. Nnadi earned a B.Sc. degree in pharmacy cum laude from Crieghton University in Nebraska in 1977; an M.Sc. degree in hospital pharmacy in 1978 from University of Minnesota; a Ph.D. degree in social and administrative sciences in 1981 from the University of Minnesota; and a J.D. degree with high honors from the College of Law at Florida State University (FSU) in 1993.

She is an experienced teacher, an accomplished researcher, and a prolific writer. At FAMU, she taught numerous courses in pharmacy administration. She was the principal or co-investigator on several grants. She has authored or co-authored several articles in professional journals and several chapters in books, and is the editor of *Health Research, Design and Methodology*, a textbook published by CRC Press.

Dr. Nnadi is an active member of several professional associations and serves on several local and national professional committees.

She has received numerous honors and awards. She was inducted into Rho Chi in 1976. At FAMU, she received the Faculty Incentive Award for Dedication and Outstanding Service in 1985, and the Golden Pen Award for the greatest number of publications in 1988. At Florida State University College of Law, she received three book awards in 1991 and 1992 for receiving the highest grades in some subjects. She graduated in the top 8 percent of her class in 1993, while carrying the full responsibilities of professor and mother. She was inducted into the Order of Coif a Law Honor Society for her achievement in law school. She is listed in *International Who's Who of Professionals* in 1996. She is also a licensed pharmacist and an attorney.

Contributors

Maxine Myers Agazie, Ph.D., A.C.S.W., is associate professor in the Department of Psychology, Sociology and Social Work at Albany State College, Albany, Georgia.

She received a B.A. degree in social studies from Benedict College, Columbia, South Carolina; an MSSW degree in social work from the University of Tennessee, Knoxville, Tennessee; and a Ph.D. in counseling from Atlanta University, Atlanta, Georgia. She was a Fulbright scholar in India.

Dr. Agazie has worked as a psychiatric social worker at Arkansas State Hospital, Benton, Arkansas; as a medical social worker at Grady Memorial Hospital, Atlanta, Georgia; as clinical director of the Substance Abuse Program at Florida Correctional Institution, Lowell, Florida; as social welfare officer with the Ministry of Health and Social Welfare, Nigeria, West Africa; and as a social work educator at universities in North Carolina, Florida, and Virginia.

Mable Smith-Pittman, R.N., Ph.D., J.D., is an associate professor in the School of Nursing at Old Dominion University in Norfolk, Virginia. She received her B.S.N. degree in nursing in 1980 from Florida State University; an M.N. in adult health nursing from Emory University in Atlanta, Georgia, in 1984; and a Ph.D. in higher education administration in 1988 and a J.D. degree in 1992 from Florida State University in Tallahassee, Florida.

Dr. Smith-Pittman has worked in various staff nurse positions. She has also served as assistant professor in the School of Nursing at Florida A&M University, and coordinator and associate professor in nursing at the University of Southern Mississippi–GP, Long Beach, Mississippi.

She has written for several professional publications and is a member of national legal and nursing professional organizations, including Phi Delta Phi Law Honorary Society, Sigma Theta Tau, the American Bar Association, the Florida Bar Association, the Virginia State Bar Association, the Virginia Trial Lawyers' Association, and the Association of Nurse Attorneys.

Anthony K. Wutoh, Ph.D., is assistant professor of clinical and administrative pharmacy sciences at Howard University College of Pharmacy and Pharmaceutical Sciences. Dr. Wutoh received a B.A. degree in biochemistry from the University of Maryland–Baltimore County in 1987. He then completed a B.S. degree in pharmacy and a Ph.D. degree in pharmacy administration (pharmacoepidemiology) at the University of Maryland School of Pharmacy. He has varied research interests, including pharmacoepidemiology, outcomes research, and evaluation of large population databases, particularly in the area of AIDS and HIV infection.

Dr. Wutoh has been a practicing pharmacist in Maryland since 1990 and has worked in hospital, retail, consulting, and community pharmacy. In 1993, he served as a policy intern with the U.S. Senate Special Committee on Aging, where he evaluated the economic impact of healthcare reform on the pharmaceutical and biotechnology industries. His other areas of interest and expertise include postmarketing assessment, clinical trial protocol and evaluation, survival analyses, and the role of stress in the functioning of healthcare professionals.

Management and Communication 1

The development of management principles has had a fairly long history. Most of the credit for developing these principles and views belongs to pioneers such as Fredrick W. Taylor,[1] originator of the scientific management style, and Henri Fayol,[2] who conceived the general and industrial administrative system. Taylor maintained that the work of management can be analyzed scientifically so as to arrive at better decisions. His scientific analysis included the following:

- Research into the nature of the variables bearing upon problems.
- Standardized application of the methods developed to all applicable jobs.
- Selection of workers in the method best suited to performing the jobs analyzed.
- Training workers in the best method developed for performing the work.

Fayol, on the other hand, conceived management as consisting of several distinct functions or processes. These include planning, organizing, commanding or directing, coordinating, and controlling.

- *Planning* includes studying the future and arranging a course of action to meet future needs. Planning is a method of achieving an organization's goals and objectives.
- *Organizing* includes gathering and building up material as well as human organization of the enterprise to meet organizational goals.

- *Commanding* or *directing* includes influencing employees to do their work.
- *Coordinating* includes uniting and correlating all activities.
- *Controlling* includes making sure that all activities are performed in line with the rules established by the organization.

Chester L. Bernard[3] emphasized the function of the leader as a dimension of studying organizational behavior. People, their interactions, and their behaviors, he emphasized, belong to a large system of social relationships of which a single organized institution is but a subsystem. The principle of efficiency as Bernard employed it encompasses such matters as individual and group satisfaction. According to Bernard, subordinates will likely consider an institutional structure to be effective if it operates without waste or carelessness and makes for work satisfaction. The work of Bernard tends to lend credence to Gilbreth's[4] advice to users of the scientific management style: The advocate must look at workers first and understand their personalities and needs.

MANAGEMENT AND HUMAN RESOURCES MANAGEMENT DEFINED

Management can be defined as the art and science of planning, organizing, commanding or directing, coordinating, and controlling tasks in an organization to achieve organizational goals and objectives.

Human resources management, also called personnel management, is that aspect of management involving human resources in an organization. Personnel or human resources management involves any and all activities that affect employees in the work environment, such as

- Employee relations
  - —Selection of employees
  - —Wages and salaries
  - —Fringe benefits and employee services
  - —Grievance procedures

- Employee development
  - —Management and other forms of employee training
  - —Personnel research
  - —Continuing education and training programs for employees

- Employee safety and health

—Safety programs in the work environment
—Frustration
—Job burnout
—Stress management

- Regulatory aspects of employee management
  —Federal fair employment practices
  —Workers' compensation
  —Employment discrimination issues
    1. Title VII
    2. The Americans with Disabilities Act (ADA)
    3. The Age Discrimination in Employment Act (ADEA)
    4. Sex discrimination
    5. The Family and Medical Leave Act (FMLA)
    6. The National Labor Relations Act (NLRA/Wagner Act)
    7. Sexual harassment

The Role of Human Resources Management in Healthcare

Any professional practice, regardless of size and organizational setup, can be successful only if it has the right type and number of individuals working in it, since the manager or owner cannot do everything. Staffing is critical in all practice settings, regardless of type or size. Individuals in administrative roles take certain risks in hiring a new employee. However, the smaller the practice, the less it is able to afford the time and costs involved in hiring a wrong employee, dismissing that employee, and hiring another.

Employees are a vital link between the services any healthcare professional offers and the patients receiving those services. Employees also play a significant role in setting the professional image and creating client loyalty. Human resources management involves recruiting, selecting, training, developing, promoting, disciplining, and dismissing employees. Large organizations such as corporations may have personnel departments that handle most of these functions; in small independent healthcare practices, however, the owners have to handle most of these personnel management issues. Therefore, skill in human resources management is essential to the small independent practitioner's success and continued survival. Poor personnel management may lead to expensive legal problems.

Also, salaries and wages represent an important portion of business expenses, and a high employee turnover rate can be expensive not only in terms of training costs but also in its negative effect on other employees. Healthcare practitioners should develop human resources policies and keep them up to date. Carefully developed policies should cover all matters affecting employees, such as salaries and wages, fringe benefits, working hours, vacation, time off, training, promotion, grievances, employee evaluation, unacceptable practices, employment termination, and retirement.

COMMUNICATION IN EMPLOYEE RELATIONS

The importance of good communication techniques in the overall management of any form of healthcare practice cannot be overemphasized. It is essential not only in employee relations but also in patient relations. Communication in some areas of the practice such as informed patient consent, must be documented.

Communication Defined

Communication can be defined as a means of transmitting or exchanging information through a medium between a sender and a receiver, with the intent of receiving a response through a feedback mechanism. The sender is the initiator of the communication process, while the receiver is the intended audience. The medium is the channel through which the communication is sent, such as paper, television, telephone, or radio.

Communication is also a means of exchanging messages or thoughts. Communication can be thought of as the process of establishing a commonness or oneness of thought between a sender and a receiver. The implied commonness of thought in this definition indicates the necessity of a sharing relationship between sender and receiver in order to achieve effective communication. Thus, both the sender and receiver should be active participants in the communication process. When a patient, because of difficulty with the language or any other reason, is unable to understand instructions given by a health professional, there will be no commonness or oneness of thought, and communication will fail.

In a case of perfect communication, if there were such a thing, all messages would be sent and received exactly as intended. However, communication is subject to interpretation, and thus lends itself to misinterpretation and misunderstanding.

Most employee problems stem from misunderstanding or misinterpretation of communicated information. Often this results from lack of feed-

back to the sender, or the lack of information in the form of an acknowledgment of what the receiver heard.

Forms of Communication

In healthcare settings, communication can take place in several forms:

- *Written communication.* In most work settings this consists of letters,
  memos, invitations, notices, announcements, policies, and procedures.
  Over time, this is a more reliable form of communication than oral
  communication.
- *Oral communication.* Oral information is more likely to be forgotten over
  a period of time than written communication. It is also more likely to
  be misinterpreted.
- *Nonverbal communication.* This is just as important as written communi-
  cation and oral communication. Nonverbal communication includes
  —Facial expressions (smiles, for example).
  —Gestures (such as use of hands or nodding).
  —Dress and general appearance.
  —Body positions and movements.
  —Body contact (touching, for example).

These types of nonverbal communication are often referred to as "body
language"; they convey attitudes and feelings.[5] The work environment
itself (whether it is clean or dirty, for example) and its decor are a form of
nonverbal communication. Both verbal and nonverbal communication
should convey the same message. Where the nonverbal communication con-
tradicts the verbal message, it reduces the credibility of what is being said.

Behavior can also communicate a message. A conflict between overt
behavior and verbal communication will create problems.[6] For example, a
healthcare practitioner or supervisor who orally or in written form tells
employees not to chew gum while working, but then either chews gum or
does not reprimand the employee who does, has nonverbally communicated approval of gum chewing or undermined the policy by demonstrat-
ing that it applies to workers but not supervisors. The supervisor is therefore transmitting conflicting messages. Often, when a nonverbal or written
message conflicts with a verbal one, the receiver is more likely to accept
the nonverbal one.[7,8] The employees in the example above might therefore
chew gum while working regardless of oral or written communication,
because there is no enforcement of the policy. This is true of most unen-
forced policies in the workplace. After a period of time, the employees will

disregard the policy, and attempts to enforce the policy without warning may create problems, including charges of discrimination.

Components of Communication

Communication has five elements, which are discussed below.

1. The *sender.* Sometimes called the source or initiator of communication, the sender is the one who has a thought to share with another. Communication therefore begins when a sender conveys a thought, experience, or feeling.
2. The *message.* This is a symbolic expression of a sender's thought. The message may be oral, written, or nonverbal. It is essential that the message be in a form that the intended audience will understand.
3. The *medium.* This is the path or mechanism though which the message is transmitted to the intended audience. The medium is also called the channel. Examples of media include radio, telephones, television, and paper.
4. The *receiver.* This is the intended audience of the message. The sender transmits the message to the receiver.
5. *Feedback.* This indicates the two-way nature of effective communication. Feedback assures the sender that the intended message is received (or that it was not received). It is also a means of clarifying information. In one-way communication, there is no feedback. Feedback, like the message, can be oral, nonverbal, or written (see figure 1).

Barriers to Effective Communication

Misunderstanding results from the following barriers to effective communication:

- Use of inappropriate vocabulary—for example, when a healthcare worker uses medical terminology unfamiliar to a patient.
- Selective attention—in which either the sender or receiver is working on something else while attempting to communicate. It also occurs when the sender or receiver is eavesdropping on another communication during the communication process.
- Failure to solicit and receive feedback—for example, when a health worker presumes that a patient understood the instructions and doesn't bother to find out whether the instructions were understood.
- Preoccupation with personal concerns—this occurs when an individual is worried or daydreaming about personal issues during communication.

Figure 1. *Communication Model*

	message	
Sender	——————————————————→	Receiver
	medium/channel	

(For example, nursing supervisor)   (For example, nursing employee)

		Receiver
interprets		interprets
feedback	feedback	message
received ◄———————————————————		and send
from message	medium/channel	feedback
received		to sender

(For example, nursing supervisor   (For example, nursing employee)

- Conflicting messages—in which verbal communication conflicts with other forms of communication.
- Inappropriate timing of information.

It is important that employers and supervisors pay attention to these barriers to effective communication in the workplace. Improved and open communication often leads to a better work environment.

In handling employee issues, one should show empathy. This means putting oneself in the other person's place, understanding the other person's point of view and where the other person is coming from.

For effective communication, it is important that the supervisor be a good listener. Listening is probably one of the most important dimensions of communication. It reduces the chance of miscommunication. Employees should be encouraged to solicit feedback to be sure that what was communicated was understood. The supevisor could ask the employee to repeat the message. Timing is also important in communication. Information may be better received at one time than another.

The medium or channel through which a message is sent is also important.[9] The choice of channel should be based on the nature of the message, whether there is a need for immediate employee feedback, and how soon employees must understand and accept the message.

Figure 2. *Horizontal Communication*

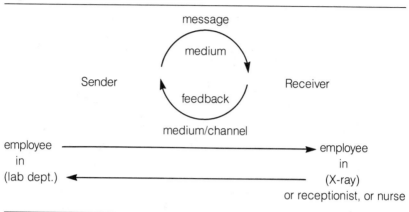

Lateral or Horizontal Communication

Communication can be lateral (horizontal) or vertical. Lateral communication involves interdepartmental transmission of information. It is horizontal because of the interdependence of people at the same level in an organization. Lateral communication is essential to coordinating activities and facilitating interaction among the various areas in any healthcare setting. In a medium-size or large medical clinic, for example, with different health professionals, such as nurses and laboratory employees, lateral communication is essential to the performance of their jobs (see figure 2).

Vertical Communication

Vertical communication involves transmission of information up and down the chain of command, such as between an employee and a supervisor (see figure 3).

With the increase in group practices and other related practice organizations such as associations and foundations, the need for both horizontal and vertical communication becomes very important. A supervisor must communicate with employees regarding their responsibilities and limitations. This is critical even in healthcare settings that use several types of aid and care extenders. Health maintenance organizations (HMOs) and managed-care organizations, which are attempting to reduce healthcare costs while maintaining quality healthcare, require good horizontal and vertical communication to function properly. As in all healthcare set-

Figure 3. *Vertical Communication*

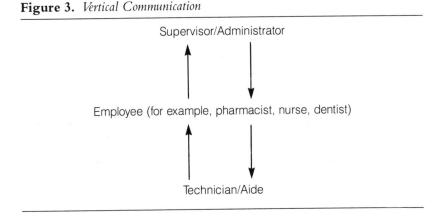

tings, effective communication is a key to successful human resources management.

CHAPTER 1 REFERENCES

1. Taylor, F.W. *Scientific Management* (New York: Harper and Brothers, 1947).
2. Fayol, H. *General and Industrial Management* (New York: Pitman Publishing Company, 1949).
3. Bernard, Chester L. *The Functions of the Executive* (Cambridge, MA: Harvard University Press, 1938).
4. Gilbreth, L. *Psychology of Management* (New York: Sturgis and Walton Company, 1914).
5. Fast, J. *Body Language* (New York: M. Evans and Company, Inc., 1970).
6. Sigband, Norman B. *Communicating for Management* (Glenview, IL: Scott, Foresman and Company, 1969).
7. Ruesch, J., and Weldon, K. *Nonverbal Communication* (Los Angeles: University of California Press, 1956).
8. Campbell, J.H., and Hepler, H.W. *Dimensions in Communication*, 2nd ed. (Belmont, CA: Wadsworth Publishing Co., Inc., 1970).
9. Melcher, A.J., and Beller, R. "Consideration in Channel Selection," *Academy of Management Journal*, 10, 1, March 1967, 39–52.

Leadership and Supervision 2

Leadership and supervision are essential to achieve organizational goals and create a good work environment to promote employee motivation and encourage desired behavior. The leader interprets, applies plans, and controls, and therefore must give these functions meaning to employees, and indicate their relevance to the tasks employees face.

The earliest tradition of leadership assumes that leaders are born and not made. Thus, anyone who is a leader was destined to become one. This is not necessarily true. In modern times, people get promoted into leadership roles. An individual graduating from a professional school with the appropriate license to practice a new profession can be hired into a managerial or supervisory position without possessing hereditary skills in leadership. For example, a newly licensed pharmacy graduate may be hired as a pharmacy supervisor. Individuals who set up their own independent practice also find themselves in leadership roles upon opening the practice; independent optometry practice, for example, is common in medical clinics, health maintenance organizations, and shopping malls. Not every one in a leadership position has the qualities to be a good leader; an individual may be hindered by personality traits, lack of experience, or the social environment. However, healthcare professionals can learn which traits are desirable in leaders, and work to acquire those qualities.

Leadership Defined

"Leadership" refers to the interpersonal process by which a healthcare supervisor tries to influence employees to perform their work. The sum total of the behavior of a supervisor, manager, owner, or executive in direct relation to subordinates and employees could be termed leadership.

Ten Characteristics and Qualities of Good Leaders

A good leader

1. Is self-motivated.
2. Adapts to change because he or she is open-minded, flexible, sees change as opportunity, and enjoys challenges.
3. Solicits input from others, thus allowing diverse opinion.
4. Is goal oriented.
5. Strives for excellence.
6. Works well with people.
7. Perseveres.
8. Delegates as appropriate.
9. Has confidence in his or her capabilities.
10. Works hard.

TYPES OF LEADERSHIP

Leadership can be people oriented or task oriented.

People-Oriented Leadership

People-oriented leadership concentrates on considering the feelings of employees and the quality of their mutual relationship. It is sometimes referred to as democratic, participative, considerate, or laissez-faire leadership. Basically, people-oriented leadership places most emphasis upon communicating with subordinates about their needs, building strong group relationships and resolving personnel problems through counseling. It also involves group discussion and group involvement in decisions on policy issues.[1]

Although employees do not make the decisions about the goals and objectives of a practice, there should be a high degree of group participation and support. The degree of democracy can be judged by the number and significance of the decisions made by the employees.[2,3] Laissez-faire management in its true sense is rarely practiced in a work environment. It means permitting employees to do what they choose with little or no restriction. In its extreme form, it seems to imply the absence of leadership.

Research as to the effects that people-oriented leadership has on productivity, group cohesiveness, and employee satisfaction seems to suggest that this form of leadership results in more positive attitudes, lower absentee rates, moderate to higher productivity, increased employee satisfaction and morale, and enhanced group cohesiveness.[4,5,6,7,8,9]

The effectiveness of participative leadership also seems to be a function of the personal characteristics of the employees. Some employees have a high need for independence, while others do not. For people-oriented leadership to be effective, participation must be perceived as sincere, not manipulative.[10]

Although there seems to be evidence that people-oriented leadership leads to increased production, it is not to say that this leadership style by itself will increase productivity. In fact, there is evidence to suggest that people oriented leadership is not consistently related to high productivity,[9,11] implying that in some situations people-oriented leadership may result in lower productivity. The success of a leadership style therefore depends on the situation. The type of leadership required in one situation may not be appropriate in another.

Task-Oriented Leadership

Task-oriented leadership, unlike people-oriented leadership, focuses on the work to be performed, and gives little attention to employee feelings. It is sometimes referred to as autocratic, directive, structured, or authoritarian management. The essence of this leadership style is an overriding concern with the task itself. It involves a high degree of direction from the manager, with little or no employee participation. Being task-oriented does not necessarily mean being harsh, however. It simply puts the work to be done, and its accomplishment, first.

There is conflicting evidence in the Management literature as to the relationship between task-oriented leadership and productivity.[12] However, this form of leadership often depresses employee satisfaction and morale.[13,14,15]

It may be best to use different leadership styles, as the situation warrants. Using a task-oriented leadership style at one point does not mean that people-oriented leadership cannot be used at another. The healthcare administrator need not be strictly task- or people-oriented. A happy medium may be found by which the task is well accomplished and employee satisfaction and morale are maintained.

SOME THEORIES ON LEADERSHIP

X and Y Theory

One of the most important leadership theories is that of Douglas McGregor, often referred to as McGregor's X and Y Theory. McGregor described two sets of assumptions, X and Y, which may lead to two different types of leadership styles. The following are the basic assumptions of Theory X:[16]

- The average human being has an inherent dislike of work and will avoid it if he can.
- Because of this human characteristic of disliking work, most people must be coerced, controlled, directed, or threatened with punishment to get them to put forth adequate effort toward the achievement of organizational objectives.
- The average human prefers to be directed, wishes to avoid responsibility, has relatively little ambition, and wants security above all.

Theory Y, on the other hand, involves a quite different set of assumptions:[17]

- The expenditure of physical and mental effort in work is as natural as play or rest.
- External control and the threat of punishment are not the only means for bringing about effort toward organizational objectives. People will exercise self-direction and self-control in the service of objectives to which they are committed.
- Commitment to objectives is a function of the rewards associated with their achievement.
- The average human being learns, under proper conditions, not only to accept but to seek responsibility.
- The capacity to exercise a relatively high degree of imagination, ingenuity, and creativity in the solution of organizational problems is widely, not narrowly, distributed in the population.
- Under the conditions of modern industrial life, the intellectual potentialities of the average human being are only partially utilized.[18]

Theory Y may lead to people-oriented leadership and to clear demands for high performance. Theory X exemplifies the traditional use of authority seen in extremely task-oriented management.

Management Grid Theory

Another important management theory was developed by Blake and Mouton. In their Management Grid, they placed leadership styles into five major categories, depending on whether the manager is task or people oriented. A manager can be

1. Highly task oriented and minimally people oriented. This type of management or leadership style shows high concern for getting the job done but shows little or no concern for employees' feelings. This typifies the manager who wants the job done no matter what it takes. Blake and Mouton refer to this as a 9,1 managerial style.
2. Minimally task oriented and highly people oriented (a 1,9 managerial style). In this instance the manager is highly concerned about people and minimal concerned about the task.
3. Highly task oriented and highly people oriented (a 9,9 management style). This management seems to increase productivity in the workplace as well as increase employee morale. The manager is not only highly concerned about getting the job done but equally concerned about how the job affects the employees.
4. Somewhat task oriented and somewhat people oriented (a 5,5 management style). In this type of management style, the manager maintains medium concern for both task accomplishment and people.
5. Minimally task oriented and minimally people oriented (a 1,1 management style). According to the Grid Theory this may lead to poor management, low productivity, and employee dissatisfaction. Therefore this form of managerial style should be avoided.

MANAGEMENT BY OBJECTIVE

Management by Objective (MBO) is closely related to employee performance evaluation. It is based on quantitative performance goals, which are set jointly by the supervisor and employee. Using this approach, the employee establishes short-term goals to improve both the employee's own efficiency and that of the organization. At the end of a set period (six months to a year), both employee and supervisor meet again to evaluate how well the set goals have been met.

Advantages

MBO has the following advantages:

- It emphasizes future accomplishments rather than dwelling on the past.
- It is a tool to measure and judge performance.
- It creates for each employee a standard of evaluation based on the special characteristics of each job.
- It aids in clarifying responsibilities and expectations for the employee and supervisor.
- It puts the supervisor in the position of coach rather than judge.
- It provides the employee with clear goals and objectives.
- It enhances communication between the employee and the supervisor.
- It helps to stimulate and motivate employees by allowing them to set their own goals and meet overall organizational goals.
- It improves employee performance because the employee has definite goals to meet in a specified period of time.
- It promotes delegation and decentralization.
- It fosters increasing employee competence and growth.
- It improves employee self-esteem and independence.

Disadvantages

Although MBO does have its advantages and can serve as an effective management style to improve employee productivity and motivation, it also has its drawbacks.

- The effectiveness of MBO depends on the supervisor's leadership style. The supervisor who is very directive and decisive may end up setting the goals and handing them down to the employee, rather than letting the employee set the goals.
- The employee may set goals to try to please the supervisor.
- The employees may emphasize only tangible, measurable performance at the expense of other important aspects of the job.
- Employees may set low, easily achievable goals in order to look good.
- It is difficult for an employee to set and achieve goals that are partly dependent on someone else's performance.

- MBO is uncomfortable for those employees who want and need to be directed. These employees would rather be told what to do than set their own goals for getting their job done.
- Spending too much time on setting goals and meeting with the supervisor takes time away from the work to be performed.

Steps in Management by Objective

There are five steps in the implementation and utilization of MBO.

1. The employee and supervisor must first discuss the employee's understanding of the job description and analysis. Each employee must know the organization's goals and how that individual's job helps achieve these goals.
2. The employee, with the help of the supervisor, establishes short-term performance goals consistent with the organizational goals. These goals should be measurable and have definite completion dates. If the goals become overly qualitative rather than quantitative, they will become difficult to effectively measure and it will be hard to determine each employee's accomplishment. However, the qualitative aspects of each job should not be ignored. A definite time period for accomplishment is also very important, and the time period must be realistic.
3. There should be regular meetings between the employee and supervisor to discuss progress toward accomplishing the goals. Identified problems are dealt with and goal adjustments are made if possible.
4. The employee and supervisor must establish checkpoints to measure progress.
5. At the end of the predetermined period, the employee and supervisor will meet to assess the employee's performance.

MBO is a useful management tool and provides a framework within which employees are motivated, know where they stand, and know what they should do to improve themselves. Goal setting by employees, when appropriately done, is more effective than goal setting by the supervisor.

Where MBO in an actual work setting deviates very much from the theory, a number of problems may occur:[19]

- Tension and anxiety about achieving goals.
- Developing inappropriate goals, just because they can be easily achieved.
- Continued pursuit of set goals when they should have been abandoned because of changed conditions.

Most of these problems arise as a result of inadequate planning and implementation of Management by Objective. With adequate planning and implementation, MBO can be a success.

STRATEGIES AND SUGGESTIONS FOR SUCCESSFUL LEADERSHIP

Although different situations require different management or leadership styles, there are some general characteristics of successful leadership:

1. Successful leaders treat their employees the way the leaders themselves would like to be treated.
2. A good leader does not ask employees to do what the leader will not do. This means leading by example. If a leader or supervisor does not want employees to be late arriving at work, then the supervisor must also be on time.
3. A leader who makes an error will admit the mistake and apologize as appropriate. This will help others to do so.
4. Good leaders avoid public criticism of individual employees because it might alienate other employees from the supervisor. However, overall criticism of work that needs improvement, or of unacceptable practices, is appropriate.
5. A good leader emphasizes the strengths of the employees in the workplace and acknowledges individuals' contributions. This makes employees feel that they are an essential part of the organization and that they are appreciated.
6. A good leader has a clear vision of the organization's direction. Vision is important, because it guides the organization. It tells employees where they are going as an organization, and why.
7. A good leader is flexible and open minded, and can adapt to changes in healthcare.
8. Successful leaders seek input from employees, especially on issues affecting the employees.

CHAPTER 2 REFERENCES

1. White, R., and Lippitt, R. "Leadership Behavior and Member Reaction in Three Social Climates," in Dorwin Cantwright and Alvin

Zander, eds., *Group Dynamics*, 2nd ed. (Evanston, IL: Row, Peterson, 1960).

2. White, R.K.; Lippitt, R., and Lewin, K. *Autocracy and Democracy: An Experimental Inquiry.* (New York: Harper & Row, 1960).

3. Tannenbaum, R., and Schmidt, W. H. "How to Choose a Leadership Pattern," *Harvard Business Review*, 36, March-April 1958, 98.

4. Tannenbaum, R., and Schmidt, W.H. "Retrospective Commentary," *Harvard Business Review*, 51, May-June 1973, 166–168.

5. Likent, R. *New Patterns of Management* (New York: McGraw-Hill, 1961).

6. Morse, N.C., and Reimer, E. "The Experimental Change of a Major Organizational Variable," *Journal of Abnormal and Social Psychology*, 52, January 1956, 120–129.

7. Coch, L., and French, J. "Overcoming Resistance to Change," *Human Relations*, 1, 1948, 512–532.

8. Kahn, R.L., and Katz, D. "Leadership Practices in Relation to Productivity and Morale," in D. Cantwright, and A. Zander, eds., *Group Dynamics*, 2nd ed. (Evanston, IL: Row, Peterson, 1960).

9. Stogdill, R.M. *Handbook of Leadership* (New York: Free Press, 1974).

10. French, John R.P., Joachim Israel, and Dagfinas, "An Experiment in Participation in Norwegian Factory," *Human Relations*, 13, February 1960, 3–19.

11. Locke, E.A., and Scheiger, D.M. "Participation Decision Making: One More Look," in Barry M. Staw, ed., *Research in Organizational Behavior*, Vol. 1 (Greenwich, CT: JAI Press, 1979), 265–339.

12. Stogdill, R.M. *Handbook of Leadership Style* (New York: Free Press, 1974).

13. Baumgartel, Howard. "Leadership Style as a Variable in Research Administration," *Administrative Science Quarterly*, 2L 344–360, December 1957.

14. Lewin, Junt, "The Consequences of an Authoritarian and Democratic Leadership," in Alvin W. Gouldner, ed., *Studies in Leadership* (New York: Harper & Brothers, 1950).

15. White, R., and Lippitt, R. Op. cit.

16. McGregor, Douglas. *The Human Side of Enterprise* (New York: McGraw-Hill, 1960).

17. Ibid.

18. Ibid.

19. Levinson, Harry. "Management by Whose Objectives"? *Harvard Business Review*: 48, 4, July-August 1970, 125–134.

Employee Selection, Training, and Assessment   3

REASONS FOR JOB VACANCIES

A position becomes available in a healthcare setting for various reasons:

Company Growth

A job opening may become available as a result of growth and expansion in the services provided. A medical clinic, for example, that provides laboratory, x-ray, or other diagnostic services may want to either expand existing clinical services or develop new services that it does not currently provide. An organization may need another healthcare professional because it is extending its hours of operation to better accommodate clients. In these instances, a new position that has not been held by any other employee becomes available.

Employee Resignation

A position may become available because an employee resigns. Reasons for employee resignation include

- Finding a better job elsewhere.
- Having to leave town with family for personal or professional reasons.
- Personality problems with other employees or management.
- Promotion into another position in the same organization.

- Health problems.
- A decision to pursue further education as a full-time student.
- Resigning to avoid dismissal.

Termination of Employment

Termination of employment is another means by which positions become available. Employees are laid off when the services they provide are no longer needed, such as during poor economic conditions, when the practice can no longer afford to keep them, or during mergers or acquisitions of one company by another. In the past, layoffs in healthcare were rare. They are becoming more frequent now as cost-reduction measures are demanded by third-party payers. Layoffs may also occur as a result of vertical or horizontal mergers of healthcare facilities. A healthcare employee can be dismissed for many reasons, such as

- Dissatisfaction with employee job performance.
- Disorderly or unprofessional conduct.
- Unlawful acts.
- Personality problems or poor manners.
- Pilferage (employee stealing).
- Excessive tardiness or absenteeism.
- Working for a competitor without permission.
- Intoxication on the job or substance abuse.
- Misrepresentation on the employment application.
- Loss of a license required to practice in the profession.

Death

The death of an employee also may create a job vacancy.

Leaves of Absence

Although a job opening may be created when an employee takes a leave of absence, such openings are usually temporary, unless the employee on leave decides not to return to work.

Retirement

Employee retirement also will usually create job vacancy.

EMPLOYEE RECRUITMENT AND SELECTION

Job Analysis

Whatever the reason for job opening, the main objective of the selection and recruitment process is to find the right person for the job. The individual responsible for hiring a new employee must determine what type of position is available—for one thing, jobs are sometimes redefined at a time of employee turnover. Will the position require special skills or special education? Can an individual be trained on the job? To find the right person, job analysis, description, and specification are essential.

Job analysis is the task of identifying the different elements and functions of a job. It involves not only listing the tasks and behaviors needed to perform the job, but also specifying the skills, knowledge, and ability required. Job analysis can be performed through a number of techniques.

- *Observation.* This can be done by watching a well-trained, skilled individual perform the job that is being analyzed—for example, watching an experienced clinician review a patient's chart. The observer will take notes while watching the clinician perform the task. The final write-up must include input from the clinician to ensure complete and accurate job analysis.
- *Interviews.* Interviewing individuals who are well trained in the job will help the person responsible for hiring a new employee find out what the job components consist of, how the job is done, and what aspects of the job must be done in a particular sequence and why.
- *Questionnaires.* Questionnaires filled out by experienced employees can be helpful in job analysis. The structure and development of the questionnaire are very important; a well-constructed questionnaire will provide adequate information about the job being analyzed.
- *Quantitative job analysis.* This involves quantification of the job and of the required employee traits and qualities. This is a more expensive technique than observation, interviews, or questionnaires.

Although there are several viable methods[1,2,3,4] for job analysis, the method used should be a function of the job being analyzed and of the major functions for that position. In preparing job analysis and descriptions, it is desirable to work with employees who have experience in the job.[5,6]

Job analysis is also relevant in equal employment opportunity (EEO) matters. Most EEO issues deal with selection, promotion, and other personnel decisions, and the way job analysis is conducted is often of primary importance in court decisions.[7]

Sound job analysis provides a job description and specifications, and eventual assessment and evaluation.

Job Description

Information obtained from the job analysis is compiled to develop the job description, which is a source of basic information for all human resource planning. The job description lists the structure, organization, and responsibilities of the job in sufficient detail to let the employee know what performance is expected. It tells both the employer and employee the job objectives and what is to be done. It not only describes the job; it also describes behaviors associated with job performance. The job description serves to inform and to remind employees about the details of their duties and also serves as a guide for improvement. It is an important tool for training new employees and for employee performance evaluation.

The benefits of job description includes:

- Avoiding confusion and providing understanding, clarification, and uniformity for the individual occupying the position.
- Providing the employee with realistic job expectations and with job satisfaction.
- Facilitating employee recruitment, selection, interviewing, training, and evaluation.
- Telling new employees what they should know and what is expected of them.

Job Specification

The terms "job specification" and "job description" are sometimes used interchangeably, however, job specification emphasizes the knowledge, experience, and intellect necessary to perform the job. Job specification is based on personal qualification obtained from the job description. For example, a job description for a technician will describe the major responsibilities and other functions in the technician's work area. The job specification will indicate the amount of experience, education, skills, licensing, and personality requirements needed to perform the job. It may also include a statement relating to employee health, safety, and comfort in the work environment. Job specification is often used extensively when advertising the job opening—during employee recruitment and selection. It is also used in establishing salary or wages for the position, based on the job market.

A job description describes the job; the job specification indicates the qualifications needed to perform the job. Thus, the job description and specification supplement and complement each other.[8] As a result, they are often confused with each other.

Once the job analysis, description, and specification are completed, but before advertising the job opening, a determination of salary or wages should be made based on available resources. This is often determined by what other employers in similar healthcare settings are paying individuals occupying similar positions. Other issues considered in setting the salary include prior experience, the length of that experience, and its relevance to the present position. It is also important to outline fringe benefits and working hours. Fringe benefits help attract and keep good employees. Fringe benefits may include discounts on items or services, free services for employees and their families, flexible hours, sick leave, personal holidays, insurance programs, pleasant working conditions, and group interaction. For some employees, fringe benefits, rather than salary, determine whether they will accept or reject a particular job offer.

EMPLOYEE SALARY AND FRINGE BENEFITS

To determine pay levels, the employer should check the rates for similar work in similar settings in the area. Such a survey of the local pay level is the best way to find out how much ought to be paid for a job. Employers can get most of the necessary information from sources such as the local Chamber of Commerce, major firms in the area, the U.S. Bureau of Labor Statistics, professional associations, colleagues, and national professional publications.

In studying pay rates in the area, employers should make sure they compare job descriptions, not just job titles, since job titles can be misleading. After an employer is satisfied that comparable positions with similar requirements for experience have been identified, the employer can compute an average pay rate for the job and enter it on a worksheet.

Employers may need to adjust the average rates somewhat to keep a sufficient difference between pay levels. The going rate for each job can then become the midpoints of the pay level ranges (the minimum and maximum rate of pay for each job). It is possible to set midpoints above or below the survey averages, based on the employer's ability to pay, the length of the work week, and the value of the benefit programs. The purpose of a pay range is to determine where the employee's pay and pay potential stand in relation to market rates for the work. It should help employers determine whether they need to make changes so that pay rates will be fair within the organization and competitive with the pay rates of similar organizations or healthcare settings in the community.

In general, a planned pay structure makes it possible to tie individual rates of pay to job performance and to contribution toward organizational goals. Employers have a general pay plan, but they do not pay in general— they pay each employee individually, so employers must consider how the plan will be administered to provide for individual pay increases.

There are several approaches for administering the pay increases within a planned pay structure:

- *Merit increases.* These are granted to recognize outstanding, superior or excellent employee performance and contributions. Merit increases are for individuals who have exceeded expectations or gone beyond the call of duty.
- *Promotional increases.* These are given to employees upon advancement to higher rank or greater responsibility.
- *Tenure increases.* These are given to employees for long-time service with the organization. They are often granted to employees after a specified number of years with an organization, such as 20, 30, or 40 years of dedicated service.
- *General increases.* These are granted to employees to keep the rate of pay competitive and to enable employees to keep up with the cost of living. They are sometimes called cost-of-living increases, because they enable employees to keep up with economic conditions such as inflation.

These approaches are the most common forms of employee pay increases, but there are many variations. Some annual increases are given for cost-of-living, tenure, or employment market reasons. Employers may use several of these pay increase methods, all of them, or a combination of them.

Pay increases should not be discriminatory. Employers should document salary increases for each employee and the reasons for the increases. This will be helpful in the event of a dispute over pay increases and to avoid employee dissatisfaction. To keep the pay plan up to date, the employer should revise it at least annually and make adjustments where necessary.

Employee compensation includes wages or salary, incentives, overtime, and benefits. Fringe benefits are compensation other than wages or salary. Fringe benefits include paid time for holidays, paid vacation time, life insurance, healthcare benefits, pension plans, Social Security benefits, tuition-reimbursement programs, disability insurance, credit unions, product or service discounts, legal assistance, and food services.

Employee compensation is one of the most difficult employee-relations issues for management. Employee benefits can help develop a stable and productive workforce, but employers must have effective cost and administrative controls. Social Security benefits, workers' compensation (some employers are exempt), and unemployment compensation, are legally required benefits that can be managed with minimal difficulty by keeping records, submitting forms to the proper authorities, and paying for the required coverage. But when choosing and managing other types of benefits, employers should get professional advice before setting up a program.

Usually as the cost of benefits increases in relation to total compensation, the direct pay cost percentage decreases. Employers often cannot recognize outstanding achievement with direct pay increases because funds for direct pay are diminishing as benefit spending gets bigger. As a result, unfortunately, the compensation differential between the mediocre employee and the outstanding achiever is narrowing. Healthcare employers, managers, and supervisors need to recognize the advantages and limitations of employee benefits and the cost impact they have on organizational operations and net profit.

Benefit costs can be analyzed by grouping them as follows:

- Legally required benefits, such as
  1. Social Security.
  2. Federal Unemployment Compensation (state requirements vary).
  3. Workers' compensation (may not be required for certain employers with very few employees). There are also state variations in coverage and benefit packages (see chapter 7).

- Optional benefits, such as
  1. Group insurance coverage (for example, health, life, disability, prescription, optical, or dental insurance).
  2. Pension plans.
  3. Employer service or merchandise discounts.
  4. Employee tuition-reimbursement programs.

5. Payment for time not worked (sick days, holidays, annual vacations, and personal leave).

Many pharmacy employers in large healthcare organizations pay for most, if not all, of the employee's life, medical, and disability insurance. The rapid escalation of benefit costs compared with direct pay has caused some healthcare employers, managers, owners, and supervisors to become more diligent in controlling these costs while maintaining better employee relations.

Employee benefits should be designed in consultation with competent employee benefits planner and manager. Employers should avoid copying other healthcare organizations when deciding whether to adopt a particular benefit, because this approach could result in the blind leading the blind. Healthcare employers need an approach that allows them to offer employee benefits designed to meet their employees' needs. For example, employees who are older or do not have the responsibility of young dependent family members will have different needs from employees who have such responsibilities. Also, employees whose spouses are employed and covered by another employer might receive benefits in such a way as to minimize double coverage. There is a trend for large employers to provide child care facilities at the workplace for the benefit of employees. The cost of such a facility may be shared by the employer and the employees using the service.

Fringe benefits are no longer merely extras, as they were once thought of. Many employees heavily rely on these benefits during illness, unemployment, retirement, vacations, holidays, and even educational and professional advancement. Collective bargaining has also contributed to the growth of fringe benefits.

Healthcare service employers provide fringe benefits to help raise employee morale. Therefore the benefits serve as a part of the motivational mechanisms the organizations create.

One of the most popular fringe benefits is group health insurance. As medical costs continue to escalate, many employees are relying on group health insurance to protect themselves and their families against high medical bills. Some healthcare organizations provide group health insurance coverage to their employees in the form of premium sharing: Both employer and employee share in the premium costs, with the employer paying a greater portion. There are, however, employers who pay all the premium costs. For some small healthcare organizations, especially small, private, independent, community-based professional practices, providing group healthcare insurance for their employees may prove challenging and expensive. Insurance companies that specialize in covering employees of small businesses can be of assistance in developing a program that may meet the needs of the healthcare employer who wishes to provide such fringe benefits for its employees.

THE EMPLOYEE SELECTION PROCESS

In recruiting new employees, it is important to consider the nature of the labor market, such as available skills. The labor market determines how long it will take to fill a particular job opening. The market can be analyzed by determining its boundaries. Qualified potential employees may be unwilling to take jobs far from their homes.

Most healthcare service organizations employ individuals with specific skills, such as licensed or registered pharmacists, nurses, dentists, and physicians. Their skills are more readily available if the workplace is located near a training site for these skills. A large dental practice, for example, that wants to hire several licensed dentists will have fewer problems if the practice is located in the same city as a school of dentistry. If a healthcare setting needs one nonprofessional employee, such as a receptionist, there will be less of a problem recruiting one even if the organization pays less than its competitors. However, to keep a good employee and reduce turnover, the organization must provide other nonfinancial incentives, such as fringe benefits.

Economic conditions will also affect employee recruitment. Although in a poor labor market with high unemployment rates employers in general are swamped by potential employees, this occurs more in the nonprofessional labor market than in the professional one. However, in times of full employment, employee recruitment may be difficult for both professional and nonprofessional personnel.

A job's attactiveness in terms of pay, fringe benefits, job security, opportunity for advancement, and the reputation of the healthcare setting will also affect employee recruitment. An employer with a poor reputation will have more difficulty attracting and keeping qualified experienced registered nurses, for example, than an employer with a good reputation. The employee selection and decision process goes through different phases (see figure 4). These phases are outlined below and discussed later.

1. Advertising the job opening

Figure 4. *Various Phases in the Employment Selection/Decision Process*

I. Advertising the job opening

II. Processing completed application forms and letters of recommendations

III. Administering tests to applicants (when approrpriate)

IV. Conducting applicant interviews

V. Making reference checks

VI. Physical examination

VII. Employment decision

VIII. Orientation and training

2. Processing completed application forms
3. Testing (when appropriate)
4. Interviewing
5. Making reference checks
6. Conducting physical examinations (where appropriate)
7. Making the employment decision
8. Orientation and training

Before advertising the job opening, it is helpful to determine the probable sources of potential employees. These sources help determine where to advertise the job opening so that the employer will be able to reach a large number of potential employees without wasting a lot of money on advertising. The seven major sources of new employees are

1. *Unemployed individuals.* These people have been laid off or discharged by another employer. An employee may be laid off or discharged because a company is going out of business, because of personality conflicts or slack times (low production), for violating a company rule, or for one of the reasons discussed earlier. It is advisable to find out the reason for unemployment before hiring a dismissed employee. An unemployed worker is often under more economic pressure to find a job than a currently employed individual. As a result the unemployed individual may be more willing to accept a job with poor working conditions than a currently employed individual; this, however, may lead to job dissatisfaction later.
2. *Currently employed individuals seeking another place of employment.* Employees who are dissatisfied with any aspect of their present employment may seek another job elsewhere. Their dissatisfaction could be related to salary, benefits, or lack of opportunity for advancement. (Various aspects of job dissatisfaction are discussed in chapter 4.)

   Individuals also may seek another place of employment because they plan to move out of the area where their present job is located.

   Economic reasons may also prompt someone who is currently employed to seek another job. The employee may need more money to meet financial responsibilities and may therefore seek a second job. In this instance, the employee has no intention of leaving the present employer but rather seeks a concurrent second job with another healthcare organization or setting.
3. *New, inexperienced employees.* These individuals are entering the workforce for the first time. They may be newly graduated from a health

professional school and have no work experience except for internships, externships, residencies, or clerkships taken during their education to acquire the needed skills. The inexperienced individual may have little or no knowledge of real world job possibilities and responsibilities in healthcare.

4. *New employees taking their first job in their new profession of healthcare.* These people are inexperienced only in their area of expertise, but not with the work in general. An example is the student completing a course of study at a health profession school who has worked in the fast-food industry or at a restaurant, gas station, cleaning business, or other non-healthcare organization while in school but upon graduation and licensure now seeks employment in the healthcare profession as a pharmacist, nurse, dentist, or physician.

5. *Raiding.* This involves attracting a key employee from a competitor. To avoid problems, it is advisable to get clearance from the present employer if trade secrets are involved. Another means of avoiding problems is to use an employment agency to make contacts for the prospective employer.

6. *Retired individuals.* This is a source that employers have only recently begun to tap. These elderly individuals are physically fit, experienced, and need an extra source of income to supplement their retirement funds. They can work part-time in nonprofessional positions, depending on their experience and expertise.

7. *Homemakers returning to the workforce.* These individuals stopped working temporarily because of family situations, most often to raise children. When the family no longer needs continuous attention, the homemakers may seek to return to work. Sometimes the family budget has become tight, making it necessary for the homemaker to return to work.

Preparing for the Search

The use of a search committee is very beneficial and highly recommended in medium-size or large organizations. The search committee should include individuals the potential employee actually will work with and should be representative of the workforce in the organization. The committee should be formed early in the search process, preferably before advertising the job opening. The committee should be actively involved in all phases of the search, including writing or reviewing the advertisement. The committee chairperson coordinates all of the committee's activities.

The committee must be given a clear indication of what it is expected to do, including the time frame for recommendation of candidates. The committee must know the job description, skills, and qualifications needed for the position to be filled.

Search committees usually serve an advisory role; they make a recommendation to someone who makes the final hiring decision. The search committee should recommend no more than four candidates and may rank them.

Advertising the Job Opening

Advertising is a mechanism for informing potential applicants of the job opening and attracting qualified potential employees. However, attracting qualified individuals is only the first step in the process of hiring new employees. The manager or person responsible for hiring must avoid hiring individuals who are either unqualified or who are unlikely to stay in the position for a reasonable time, since replacing them would be expensive. The major objective of the selection process is to screen out persons who do not adequately fit the job requirements and the overall goals of the organization. There are various means of advertising a job opening, but the key is to advertise in a medium that will reach and attract several qualified persons with the characteristics the employer needs. Advertising in the wrong medium may result in

- A lack of job applicants or an insufficient pool of qualified applicants.
- Attracting unqualified or inappropriate individuals.
- Wasting advertising dollars and getting poor results.
- Employer frustration.
- Excessive workloads on current personnel because of the employer's inability to find the right individual(s).
- Lowering standards or employee qualifications for the job, with the inherent risk of providing poor service, in an attempt to fill the job opening.

The various means of advertising for a job opening in a healthcare setting includes newspapers, government and private employment agencies, professional journals and publications, professional newsletters, the Internet, word of mouth and telephone calls, schools, billboards, colleagues, window signs, unions, radio, and television. In fact, any medium to inform potential candidates of the job opening is an advertising medium. These media are discussed below.

Figure 5. *Sample Want Ad*

DELIVERY PERSON WANTED*

Doe Home Health Care, Inc., needs a dependable person to work full time (flexible hours) as a driver. Individual must be an excellent driver, have excellent driving record, and know the city well. The individual will be responsible for delivering medications and healthcare products to customers. Doe Home Health Care, Inc., will provide delivery vehicle. References are required. If interested, see John Doe, 3 p.m. to 7 p.m. Application deadline December 12, 19   . No phone calls, please.

                                        Doe Home Health Care, Inc.
                                        200 Big Street
                                        Yourtown

---

*Please note that this sample advertisement can be placed in print media, on the radio or on television, or on the Internet. If the organization has a very limited employee advertising budget, the advertisement can be shortened to meet the employer's needs.

Newspaper advertisements. Advertisements can be placed in the "Help Wanted" or "Business" section of the newspaper. Newspaper advertisements usually attract applicants of highly variable quality, however. The advertisement should be brief and clearly indicate the position, qualifications, duties, hours to be worked, and some fringe benefits if possible. The size of the advertisement should depend on the job and the amount of money available for advertising. The advertisement should run long enough to ensure that all eligible candidates will see it. Figure 5 shows a sample advertisement by a home healthcare company looking for a delivery person.

The advertisement should also indicate the type of response desired from applicants—that is, whether they should call, come to the healthcare setting, or write in response to the job opening. If the organization expects a heavy turnout of applicants, it is advisable to discourage applicants from calling because a flood of calls would disrupt work. Applicants may be asked to come in and complete an application or to request an application in writing. This is especially important in small practice settings with a limited number of personnel.

Blind advertisements can also be used when the healthcare organization does not want to be identified. In blind advertisements, the employer often

Figure 6. *Sample Blind Ad*

PHARMACY CASHIER WANTED

A local community pharmacy needs an experienced, dependable full-time cashier. The individual will be responsible for checking customers out through the cash register, answering phones, some accounting, and other duties as assigned. The individual must have a pleasant personality, be able to work with the public, have at least one year of cash register experience, and have a high school diploma. If interested, please send your resume with names of three references before April 2, 19 , to

Box 314BA
Your Hometown Newspaper
Yourtown, State, Zip Code

---

uses a box number in care of the newspaper. Prospective employees are requested to send information (a resume, for example) rather than come to or call the facility. Blind advertisements generate fewer responses, because most prospective employees like to know who the employer is. Blind advertisements are often used for positions that do not require highly specialized technical skills. A sample blind ad is given in Figure 6.

Professional journals and newsletters. If a healthcare organization is seeking a registered or licensed healthcare professional or technician, the position should be advertised in appropriate national, state, and local association journals and newsletters, and at the local health profession school, in addition to the local newspaper. These are excellent advertising media because they target the health professional.

The Internet. This is a growing medium for advertising job openings. As more people become connected to the Internet, it will become a major source of getting information out to potential employees.

Word of mouth. Recommendations from friends, colleagues, current employees, clients and relatives are another advertising medium. When word of mouth is used, it should be emphasized that the selection process will be fair and based on the applicants' qualifications. This is important to avoid personnel problems. One disadvantage to word-of-mouth recruiting is that it may lead to nepotism, especially in supervisory positions. This may cause resentment and reduce morale among other employees, especially in medium and large healthcare organizations such as institutional practices.

Government employment agencies. State employment agencies provide free services to both employers and prospective employees and therefore serve as a means of advertising a job opening. These agencies have access to statewide and nationwide networks of job opportunity information sources and can provide their clients with a wide variety of services. Most of these agencies will screen potential employees before sending them to the healthcare organization for an interview.

Private employment agencies. Some private employment agencies do not specialize in specific occupations and skills, while others concentrate on professional healthcare employment. Specialized executive recruiting agencies are available to recruit for chief executive positions.

Private employment agencies charge for their services. Their fees may be paid by the employer or the hired employee, or by both. While some agencies base their fees on a specified, constant amount, others charge a percentage of the salary of the hired employee. If the fee is based on a percentage of salary, the higher the salary paid the employee, the higher the fee paid to the employment agency.

Local health professional schools. Various healthcare companies interview graduating senior students of health professional schools. This often takes place through the school's placement office. This recruiting method gives the employer an opportunity to screen candidates and select some for further consideration. This is the best way to attract qualified candidates and possibly hire the individual at the top of the graduating class. Such employees can bring innovative ideas to the workplace.

Billboards. This is another way to get the word around and is good when a very large number of nonprofessional jobs are opening in a large organization.

Competitors. Sometimes other people who own or manage practices similar to that of the employer can be helpful in the selection process, especially when the employer is starting a new practice. When using this source, it is important to talk only to those competitors with whom the new employer has a good relationship. Most healthcare professionals maintain good relationships with one another and are supportive of each other.

Window signs. These are especially useful for nonprofessional positions that require no experience or special training. Window signs will attract people who live in the area where the job opening is available or who walk or drive by.

Radio. This can be used to fill a job opening, but, considering the audience and the cost, it is not a good medium for advertising professional jobs. It may be effective for filling a large number of nonskilled positions in a large healthcare organization, such as a hospital, a managed care organization, or a health maintenance organization. When an organization is new to an area and hiring hundreds of employees in various capacities, radio may be an appropriate advertising medium.

Television. Television is not cost-effective except where a large number of employees are needed in a large organization, such as a new hospital. A hospital with a critical shortage of personnel could mention its need during regular advertising of its services.

Unions. This is another means of attracting qualified, experienced employees if the job opening is unionized. However, employers, particularly in small healthcare settings, who do not want union involvement will not want to use this source of filling a job opening.

Temporary employment agencies. This is a means by which a healthcare organization can temporarily meet a personnel need. In this case, the employee—a nurse, for example—is not employed by the hospital but by the agency. The hospital pays the agency, and the agency pays the nurse.

It is up to the employer to select the advertising medium that will provide the maximum exposure to potential employees without overspending on advertising. Advertising in the wrong media will only waste money and time in the search for new employees.

The Application Form

The applicant for a job opening should be required to fill out an application form. This form should be developed before advertising the job opening. It should help screen out unqualified candidates and be made available to applicants as they respond to the advertisement. A healthcare organization can develop two types of application forms—one for professional positions and another for nonprofessional positions—or one general application form for all positions (see figure 7 for a sample).

Often the application form can provide useful insights to personal traits of the applicants. An incomplete, illegible, or stained application form is an indication of potential poor performance.

Figure 7. *Sample Employment Application*

APPLICATION FOR EMPLOYMENT
NAME OF PRACTICE
ADDRESS
PHONE #:

PERSONAL

Name (last name, first name) _____

Other names you have used _____

Address _____

_____

Home address (if different from above) _____

Phone (home) _____ (work) _____

Social Security No. _____

Drivers License No. _____ State _____

Position desired _____

Full time _____ Part time _____ Temporary _____

What hours will you be available to work? From _____ to _____

Dates available for employment _____

Let us know if you have special needs by calling _____

If any of your relatives are employed here, give their name(s), department(s), and relationship to you _____

_____

EDUCATION (Please give name, address, major, degree received)

High school _____

Address _____

Dates attended _____ Date graduated _____

College _____

Address _____

Dates attended _____

Major _____ Degree received _____

Health professional school _____

Address _____

Dates attended _____

Major _____ Degree received _____

Figure 7. *Sample Employment Application (Continued)*

Graduate school _____

Address _____

Dates attended _____

Major _____ Degree received _____

Other _____

Address _____

Dates attended _____

Major _____ Degree received _____

Typing speed (if applying for clerical position) _____

FOR HEALTHCARE PROFESSIONALS AND PARAPROFESSIONALS ONLY

Are you currently licensed in this state? Yes ____ No ____ If not, when will you get a license? _____

If yes, license number _____ Date licensed _____

List other states where you are licensed _____

Has your license ever been suspended or revoked? No ____ Yes ____

If yes, explain _____

FOR DELIVERY PERSON

Do you have a current driver's license? Yes ____ No ____ If yes, what class? __

When did you start driving (year) _____

Date license obtained _____

Driver's license number _____

Has your driver's license ever been suspended or revoked? Yes ____ No ____

If yes, explain _____

Have you ever been charged with driving under the influence of alcohol or drugs? Yes ____ No ____

EMPLOYMENT EXPERIENCE

Please list your employer, starting with the most recent job.

1. Name and address of employer _____

_____

Position held _____

Dates of employment, from month/year _____ to month/year ____

Name of supervisor and phone number _____

_____

Duties performed _____

_____

Reasons for leaving _____

_____

Figure 7. *Sample Employment Application (Continued)*

2. Name and address of employer _____

   _____

   Position held _____
   Dates of employment, from month/year _____ to month/year _____
   Name of supervisor and phone number _____

   Duties performed _____

   Reasons for leaving _____

3. Name and address of employer _____

   _____

   Position held _____
   Dates of employment, from month/year _____ to month/year _____
   Name of supervisor and phone number _____

   Duties performed _____

   Reasons for leaving _____

4. Name and address of employer _____

   _____

   Position held _____
   Dates of employment, from month/year _____ to month/year _____
   Name of supervisor and phone number _____

   Duties performed _____

   Reasons for leaving _____

5. Name and address of employer _____

   _____

   Position held _____
   Dates of employment, from month/year _____ to month/year _____

Figure 7. *Sample Employment Application (Continued)*

Name of supervisor and phone number _____

Duties performed _____

Reasons for leaving _____

REFERENCES
Give names of three individuals who have worked with you whom we may
contact for references.

1. Name _____ Title _____
   Company name _____
   Address _____

   Phone _____
   Relationship to you (e.g., colleague) _____
2. Name _____ Title _____
   Company name _____
   Address _____

   Phone _____
   Relationship to you (e.g., colleague) _____
3. Name _____ Title _____
   Company name _____
   Address _____

   Phone _____
   Relationship to you (e.g., colleague) _____

Conviction of a crime does not automatically prevent employment.
Circumstances will be considered. Have you ever been convicted of any
crime? No ____ Yes ____
If yes, state crime(s) and explain _____

Figure 7. *Sample Employment Application (Continued)*

I declare that the answers given to all the questions in this application are complete and accurate to the best of my knowledge, and that any falsification, misrepresentation, or omission may result in dismissal. Unless otherwise indicated, I also authorize the verification and/or investigation of information on this application form, including contacting former employers.

Applicant's signature _____ Date _____

(Name of organization) is an equal opportunity, equal employment employer.

There is certain information an application form should not solicit, however. It should be carefully constructed to avoid any semblance of discrimination by sex, race, ethnic background, religion, birthplace, or political preference. Seeking such information in an interview is forbidden as well. Figure 8 provides a guide to questioning applicants for employment.

When hiring, employers must not misuse the information obtained from the application form. The Civil Rights Act of 1964 prohibits discrimination in employment practices because of race, religion, sex, or national origin. Public Law 90-202 prohibits discrimination on the basis of age with respect to individuals who are at least 40 but less than 70. Federal laws also prohibit discrimination against the physically handicapped. Chapter 7 discusses the legal aspects of human resources management, including employment discrimination.

When an applicant has had work experience, references not related to work may not be very important. However, if an applicant's work experience is limited, objective information may be obtained from school counselors and teachers. Personal references should be carefully considered, since applicants usually list only people who will give them a good recommendation. In addition, some references may be unwilling to give a bad written recommendation for fear that the applicant may institute a legal action against them.

Tests

Employment tests serve as a mechanism for the employer to measure individual characteristics such as honesty, manual dexterity, clerical skills, computer skills, intelligence, mental maturity, and perforamnce of sample job tasks. Performance tests, intelligence tests, aptitude tests, interest tests, and personality tests all may be helpful. Tests are used less often in small,

Figure 8. *Questioning Applicants for Employment*

A Guide for Application Forms and Selection Interviews
The general rule is that all questions asked during the selection process must be related to the performance of the job duties and responsibilities.

Inquiries	Lawful	Unlawful Before Hiring
1. Name	A. Name	A. Inquiry into any information that indicates, race, color, religion, sex, or national origin. B. Inquiry into original name of an applicant whose name has been changed by court order, or inquiry into maiden name of a woman.
2. Address	A. Inquiry into length of current and previous addresses.	A. Specific inquiry into addresses that would indicate national origin. B. Asking whether applicant owns or rents home.
3. Age	A. Asking whether applicant is between 18 and 70 years of age. If the applicant is not between 18 and 70, asking the applicant's age. B. Requiring proof of age by birth certificate after hiring.	A. Requiring birth certificate. B. Requiring baptismal record before hiring, except for religious organizations where it is a required bona fide occupational qualification for the job (for example, when hiring a Catholic priest for a hospital chapel). Asking how old applicant is.

Figure 8. *Questioning Applicants for Employment (Continued)*

Inquiries	Lawful	Unlawful Before Hiring
4. Birthplace or national origin		A. Any inquiry into place of birth or national origin. B. Any inquiry into place of birth or national origin of parents, grandparents, or spouse. C. Any inquiry into applicant's, parents', spouse's lineage, ancestry, descent, parentage, or mother tongue.
5. Race or color		A. Any inquiry that would indicate race or color.
6. Sex		A. Any inquiry that would indicate sex. B. Questions on height or weight unless employer can prove them necessary requirements for the job to be performed.
7. Religion or creed	Inquiry as to observance of religious holidays if they would create a conflict relative to the established normal work week; employer must verify undue hardship and need for unreasonable accomodation.	A. Any inquiry to indicate religion, identify denomination, customs, or religious holidays observed, unless a bona fide occupational qualification (for example, hiring a Catholic priest for a hospital chapel).

Figure 8. *Questioning Applicants for Employment (Continued)*

Inquiries	Lawful	Unlawful Before Hiring
8. Citizenship	A. Inquiring whether applicant is a U.S. citizen. B. If not, inquiring whether applicant intends to become one. C. Inquiring whether applicant is a U.S. resident. D. Inquiring whether applicant's spouse is a citizen. E. Requiring proof of citizenship, work permit, or residency before hiring.	A. Inquiring whether applicant is native born or naturalized. B. Inquiring whether parents or spouse are native born or naturalized.
9. Photographs	Requiring after hiring for identification purposes.	Requesting applicant's photograph before hiring.
10. Education	A. Inquiry into what academic professional, or vocational schools applicant attended. B. Inquiry into language skills, such as reading and writing of foreign languages.	A. Any inquiry into the nationality, or the racial or religious affiliation of a school. B. Inquiry as to mother tongue or where foreign language ability was acquired, unless necessary for job.
11. Relatives	A. Inquiry into name, relationship, and address of person to be notified in case of emergency. B. Asking names of relatives employed by the organization.	A. Any inquiry about a relative that is unlawful to ask about the applicant.

Figure 8. *Questioning Applicants for Employment (Continued)*

Inquiries	Lawful	Unlawful Before Hiring
	C. Asking names and addresses of parents or guardian of minor applicant.	
12. Organization	A. Inquiry into professional organization memberships or other memberships, excluding any organization the name or character of which indicates the race, color, sex, religion, national origin, or ancestry of its members. B. Indirect inquiry into prohibited inquiries. C. Asking what offices are held, if any in the organizations in item 12A.	Inquiry into *all* clubs, lodges, and organizations that the applicant is a member of, especially if such information would in any way indicate race, religion, color, sex, national origin, ancestry, or other prohibited inquiries.
13. Military	A. Inquiry into Military service in U.S. B. Asking what rank attained. C. Asking relationship of military experience to the position applied for. D. Requiring military discharge certificate after hiring.	A. Requesting military service records. B. Asking type of discharge.
14. Work schedule	A. Any question that is job related or has direct reflection on the job applied for.	A. Any inquiry into willingness to work any particular religious holiday.

Figure 8. *Questioning Applicants for Employment (Continued)*

Inquiries	Lawful	Unlawful Before Hiring
15. Other qualifications	A. Inquiry into willingness to work the job's schedule.	A. Any inquiry not related to the job that may suggest information permitting unlawful discrimination.
16. References	A. Requesting general personal and work references not relating to race, color, religion, sex, national origin, or ancestry.	A. Requesting references specifically from clergy unless a bona fide occupational qualification or other persons who might reflect race, color, religion, sex, national origin, or ancestry of applicant.
17. Marital and family status		A. Any inquiry into marital status, number of children, child care arrangements, or pregnancy, or inquiry that may result in limitation of job opportunity.
18. Handicaps	A. Asking whether there are any job duties the applicant cannot perform because of an impairment or a physical or mental handicap.	A. Any inquiry into applicant's disability, or disease that has been treated or is being treated, or such inquiry relating to a family member.
19. Language	A. Asking whether applicant reads, writes, or speaks a foreign lan-	A. Any inquiry into how applicant acquired fluency in a language

Figure 8. *Questioning Applicants for Employment (Continued)*

Inquiries	Lawful	Unlawful Before Hiring
	guage fluently if necessary for the job.	that may indicate natural origin.
20. Arrests and convictions	A. Asking whether applicant was ever convicted of a crime. If so, when, where, and disposition of the offense.	A. Inquiring whether applicant has ever been arrested. B. Using any arrest record to deny employment, unless the employer has proof of business/job necessity.

Notes:

1. Employers acting under approved affirmative action programs or acting under orders of equal employment law enforcement agencies of federal, state, or local governments may be exempt from some of the prohibited inquiries listed above, to the extent that these inquiries are required by such programs, agreements, or orders.
2. Employers having federal defense contracts may be exempt to the extent that otherwise prohibited inquiries are required by federal law for security purposes.
3. An inquiry is forbidden that, although not specifically listed above, is designed to elicit, in violation of the law, information as to race, color, religion, sex, national origin, or ancestry.
4. Please note that the above list should serve as a guide, and that some state laws may prohibit additional inquiries, such as sexual orientation of an applicant.

independent practices and are more common in large work settings such as industries and government. The polygraph test is used most often in dealing with theft, and not in hiring.[9] It is advisable to make sure that any test used for employee selection not only conforms to government standards and regulations, but meets the employer's needs in selecting the right employee.

Interviews

An interview is one of the most important tools in employee selection. It is most productive when the interviewer adequately prepares for it. The interview not only helps the employer hire the most suitable individual, it also helps potential employees determine whether the work environment is right for them. The effective interview involves two-way communication.

The interview can be structured, nonstructured, or a combination of both. The structured interview adheres closely to a detailed set of questions listed on a specially prepared form. Each position has a set of questions that are most appropriate for it. Figure 9 suggests items for a structured interview of a healthcare professional.

Sometimes the interviewer looks primarily for negative information rather than positive evidence of job potential. The interviewer may tend to rate interviewees who are like the interviewer higher than those who are different. The validity of interviews in selecting the best candidate for a job opening is higher when the interview process is structured than when it is unstructured and when the interviewer is looking for specific job-related elements from the applicant's work history and experience rather than seeking to assess the interviewee's psychodynamics. In a purely non-structured or nondirected interview, the interview focuses entirely on the feelings expressed by the person being interviewed and rarely relies on specific questions. The interviewee, rather than the interviewer, may therefore control the unstructured interview. Most job interviews use a combination of structured and nonstructured interviews, with more structure than nonstructure.

For an interview to be most effective, it must have an interview evaluation form (a sample is provided in figure 10). The form should reflect the skills, experience, and qualifications required in a particular job. If certain characteristics are more important, those should be given the most weight.

The interviewer should pay attention to nonverbal communication such as posture, body movements, and eye contact. The interviewer should take notes recording the responses given by the potential employee. If the applicant does not answer a question, it is best to repeat the question courteously. Do not let the applicant control the interview.

An applicant should be given the opportunity to ask questions. The questions may provide useful insight about the applicant. If an applicant is obviously not suitable for the job, the interview should not be unnecessarily prolonged.

Reference Checks

It is a good practice to check with the applicant's previous employers to learn about personal characteristics and previous job performance. To make sure that important questions get asked, it is helpful to use a checklist when making reference checks (a sample checklist is provided in figure 11). Reference checks are usually made by telephone, less frequently by

Figure 9. *Suggested Items for a Structured Interview of a Healthcare Professional*

___

Explain to Applicant

1. Duties and degree of personal judgment required.
2. Overall work environment.
3. Overall organization of the healthcare setting.
4. Answers to applicant's questions.
5. When decision to hire will be made.

Inquire of Applicant

1. Why should you be hired for this position?
2. What do you like most about your present job, and what do you like least?
3. Why would you be willing to leave your current position and come to this one?
4. From what you know about this position, what short- and long-term challenges will you face, and how will you deal with them?
5. What do you think a healthcare professional in this position should be? If you were filling this job, what qualities would you look for in an applicant?
6. What are your professional goals for self-development and improvement within the next two years?
7. What additional training do you think you will need to fully carry out the duties of this position?
8. For what are you most criticized?
9. What do you think your supervisor will say about your work performance if I call?
10. What has been the most stressful event or the most difficult aspect of your job as a healthcare practitioner? How did you deal with it?
11. Who in your current or past employment did you get along with least well, and how did you deal with it?
12. What do you consider your most important achievement as a healthcare professional?
13. What is the most difficult decision you have had to make recently? How did you deal with it?
14. What are two things you would like to avoid on your next job?
15. What type of work problems seem to create the most stress for you?
16. What is your ideal working situation?
17. What is your ideal supervisor like?
18. (Include other questions on specific skills needed for the job, given the environment.)

___

Figure 10. *Sample Interview Evaluation Form*

Name of applicant _____ Social Security # _____

Position applied for _____ Date of interview _____

Evaluated characteristics		Ratings		
(also provide comments	0	1	2	3
on rated characteristics)	poor or below average	average	good	excellent

Rating   Comments

_____ Qualifications _____

_____ Experience (if needed) _____

_____ Management experience (if needed) _____

_____ Appearance _____

_____ Aggressiveness _____

_____ Friendliness _____

_____ Potential (ability for personal and professional growth) _____

_____ Desire to work in this practice setting _____

_____ Weekend and holiday availability _____

_____ Willingness to work overtime _____

_____ Ability to work with figures _____

_____ Communications (ability to express oneself) _____

_____ Ability to get along with others _____

_____ Trustworthiness _____

_____ General presentation of self _____

_____ Enthusiasm _____

_____ Ability to work independently _____

_____ Professional organization membership (if applicable) _____

_____ Other special characteristics, qualifications, or qualities _____

_____ TOTAL POINTS (POSSIBLE MAXIMUM POINTS) = _____

COMMENTS _____

_____

_____

Recommendation: Hire _____ Reject _____ Put on reserve _____

Interviewer _____ Signature _____ Date _____
          Print name

Figure 11. *Reference Checklist*

Applicant's name _____

Position being applied for _____

Person contacted _____ Date _____

Name of organization _____

Title of individual(s) contacted _____

Why did the applicant leave? _____

Would you rehire the applicant? If not, why? _____

For how long was the applicant an employee? _____

How well did the applicant get along with other employees? _____

How well did the applicant get along with supervisor(s)? _____

Is the applicant trustworthy? _____

Dependable? _____

What was the applicant's biggest problem at work? _____

_____

What was the applicant's greatest achievement? _____

_____

_____

What was the applicant's absenteeism record? _____

_____

Is there other job-related information about the applicant that would be helpful

in making the hiring decision? _____

_____

Individual completing reference checklist:

Name _____ Signature _____ Date _____
      (Print)

_____

mail or in person. However, reference checks for high-level executive positions are often made in person.

The opinions of previous employers can be helpful in providing a well-rounded overview of an applicant's potential performance, as long as the information is truthful. Caution should be exercised when a reference check is obtained from a friend or family member of the applicant, since such references may tend to provide only positive information, and these sources may be biased.

Credit rating organizations may provide information on an applicant's character, pattern of paying bills, general reputation, and so on. Such reports are now governed by the Fair Credit Reporting Act: The applicant must be notified in writing that the information is being sought,[10] and the applicant is entitled to full disclosure from the reporting agency.[11] The applicant's driving record may indicate use of alcohol or drugs while driving.

Physical Examinations

Some employers require that an employee receive a physical examination to certify that the employee's health and physical condition match the requirements of the job. The physical examination performed by a physician may help to avoid compensation claims for an injury that actually occurred prior to employment. Health insurance costs increase when employee use of healthcare services is high, so employers may wish to avoid permitting compensation for improper claims.

Please note that an employer may not discriminate against physically handicapped or impaired persons. Employers must make reasonable accommodation for them.

The Employment Decision

Once the decision to hire a person is made, the person should be contacted to review the job requirements, salary, fringe benefits, working hours, and probationary period. If the applicant accepts the terms of the employment offer, an employment contract specifying the employment conditions must be signed by both the employer and employee, especially the employee. It is important that the applicant understand the terms of the contract and agree to them in writing. There should be a probationary period for all new employees, stated in writing.

A probationary period is a tryout time for both the employer and the employee. It usually lasts about 90 days but may last more than a year.

While the employee is paid during this period, there may not be fringe benefits. If the employee's performance proves unacceptable, the employer will terminate the employment. This should be indicated in a policy and procedure manual.

ORIENTATION AND TRAINING

It is important to get the employee off to a good start through an orientation process. A new employee should be gradually and carefully introduced into the job, and receive a written job description.

Orientation

The orientation process acquaints the new employee with the organization's goals and objectives, with its policies, and with other employees. It is a period of socialization for the new employee into the work environment.[12,13,14] Proper employee orientation will help to reduce employee anxiety, such as fear of not performing well on the job, and will increase the employee's ability to cope with the new environment.

Good employee orientation will also reduce the turnover rate among new employees.

The new employee is slowly introduced to the new position, the job expectations, and how he or she fits into the organization's overall goals and objectives.[15,16] Orientation helps the new employee to develop positive attitudes toward the organization and toward the other employees as well as to achieve job satisfaction.

During orientation, the supervisor or manager should show the new employee around, introduce him or her to other employees, and explain job performance expectations. Orientation schedules vary from informal to formal; the former is seen in small organizations and the latter in large ones. It is helpful to have a checklist to be sure nothing is left out during the orientation program.

The new employee should be provided with an employee handbook if the organization has one. The handbook should contain policies on employment issues such as sexual harassment, grievance procedures, and use of organizational resources for personal use. The employee should sign for the handbook to avoid later disputes over receipt of information contained in the handbook.

Training

In most healthcare settings, new professional employees come well equipped with most of the knowledge and skills needed to begin work. Nonprofessional personnel may require more extensive training in the healthcare environment. Training should be specifically tailored to the procedures that are intended to foster learning among employees and to achieve the goals and objectives of the organization. In community settings, the most common forms of training are on-the-job training, conference or discussion, internship, and externship. Apprenticeship was used before the development of formal training for healthcare professionals. It was a precursor of modern internships, externships, clerkships, and residencies. These forms of training are discussed further below.

On-the-Job Training

This is sometimes referred to as job instruction training. In on-the-job training, new employees receive training while actually performing their jobs; it provides job experience under working conditions. This is the most common form of training among nonprofessional or paraprofessional personnel. On-the-job training generally involves certain steps:

1. Explaining to the employee in detail the what, when, how, and why of the job.
2. Performing the job so that the employee can observe and ask questions.
3. Having the employee actually perform the job.
4. Providing immediate feedback as to how the employee performed.

The evaluation should indicate areas of excellence and areas needing improvement. Small mistakes should not go uncorrected, or the new employee may not regard them as mistakes but as acceptable practice.

Conference or Discussion

This method of individualized instruction primarily involves communication of ideas and procedures. It is often used with professional personnel. The conference or discussion method of training can be formal or informal, depending on the size or organization.

Clerkship, Externship, Internship, and Residency

The terms "externship" and "internship" have been used as if they were interchangeable, because they both provide practical experience to students outside the didactic classroom environment, although some health professional schools differentiate between these terms. Some schools have clerkship programs in addition to externships and internships, while others have only one or two of these professional practice experience programs.

Both externships and clerkships are often a part of a school's curriculum, and are required of all students. They are required courses, and students pay tuition for them. Both are usually taken for credit, and students usually are not paid during these training programs. Both programs provide opportunities for students to learn to practice their profession outside the classroom. Although clerkships are often clinically oriented, especially in pharmacy education, externships may not be.

Internships are often closely associated with licensure requirements, especially in pharmaceutical education. Before taking the licensing examination upon graduation from a professional school, the individual must have completed a certain number of hours of professional experience at a site approved by the state board. Internship training can be obtained before or after graduation, depending on the professional school's curriculum structure. At schools where internship is not part of the curriculum, it is not a prerequisite for graduation, compared to externship and clerkship, which are completed while the student is still in school. Both externship and internship use the discussion or conference method.

Internship, unlike clerkship or externship, provides a broad professional experience to the students; clerkship is purely clinical experience. Internship may have several components, such as clinical, administrative, research, and distributive functions, depending on what the state board accepts. Internship is often under the control of the state board for the profession, so schools that include internship in their curriculum must comply with state board requirements. Externships and clerkships are under the sole control of the professional school in which the student receives academic credit, but the state board may choose to grant credit for some of these hours toward internship. One major advantage of building internships into a school's curriculum is that students are eligible to take the board exam as soon as they graduate.

Residency, unlike the other professional experience programs, is not part of student training prior to being licensed as a health professional. Residencies are specialty training programs for new health professionals who wish to specialize in an area such as pediatrics or psychiatry. Residents are often licensed in their profession while going through the residency program, which lasts from one to several years. Medium to large healthcare organizations may have interns, externs, and residents receiving training.

Corporate Training Programs

These are formal company programs through which new employees, especially health professionals, are informed of company policies and procedures. These programs are used in large corporations in the healthcare industry.

JOB EVALUATION AND ASSESSMENT

New employees should be evaluated after their training to determine the effectiveness of the training and to assess what learning has actually occurred. Job evaluation should be an ongoing process and not be limited to new employees.

Job evaluation is the process of grading and judging an employee's performance in relation to the work. Most procedures for evaluating employee job performance involve some form of rating scales[17,18,19,20,21] (figure 12 provides an example).

Employee job evaluation serves several functions, for example,

- Determines whether a new employee is performing the job appropriately.
- Serves as a tool for employee promotion.
- Provides an opportunity for job enrichment and improvement.
- Lets employees know how well they are performing and whether they are meeting or exceeding organizational expectations.
- Encourages and reinforces good working habits.
- Discourages poor and unsafe working habits.
- Provides a basis for disciplinary action and eventual dismissal if necessary.

Employees should be evaluated on a regular basis. It is best to conduct evaluations twice a year, but once a year is better than no evaluation. New employees should be evaluated at the end of their probation period and again after six months. During employee evaluation, it is very important that the supervisor or manager adhered to certain rules.

Figure 12. *Employee Performance Rating Scale*

Rating	Poor[1]	Fair[2]	Good[3]	Excellent[4]	Not Applicable
1. Dependability					
2. Quality of work					
3. Job knowledge					
4. Ability to work with others					
5. Ability to work independently					
6. Courteousness					
7. Communicates well with patients					
8. Communicates well with others (non-patients)					
9. Creativity					
10. Professionalism					
11. Alertness					
12. Shows concern to others					
13. Cleanliness					
14. Enjoyment of the job					
15. Professional development activities, involvement, etc.					
16. Initiative					
17. Being on time to work					

[1]Needs improvement. Does not meet minimum requirements.
[2]Meets job requirements.
[3]Exceeds job requirements.
[4]Far exceeds job requirements.

The Evaluation Process

To avoid missing an essential part of the evaluation and to make the evaluation effective, it is important for the evaluator to follow these seven steps:

1. Inform the employee of the purpose or function of the evaluation.
2. Perform the evaluation using a rating scale (see figure 12).
3. Encourage the employee to make general comments on the evaluation and the process.
4. Give the employee an opportunity to indicate any problems in relation to the job and suggest how these can be solved.
5. At the end of the evaluation, inform the employee of apparent strong and weak points and how the weak points can be strengthened. Anticipate possible hostility or aggression from the employee, especially if there are personality conflicts between the employee and the evaluator.
6. After the evaluation has been rated or scored, inform the employee of his or her performance. Allow the employee to make comments about the evaluation. Be prepared: These might be negative, defensive, or hostile.
7. Have the evaluation signed and dated by both evaluator and employee. The employee signature should indicate acknowledgment that the evaluation was done, not necessarily agreement with the rating.

Basic Principles of Employee Evaluation

It is important to follow these eight basic principles for an effective performance evaluation. Ignoring the principles will create problems such as employee dissatisfaction and frustration. It may also turn evaluation from a tool for improving the workplace into a source of anxiety for both employees and supervisors.

1. Employee evaluation should not be kept a secret. The employee should know the criteria for the evaluation and when the evaluation will occur. The employee should also know who will perform the evaluation. If the employee will be evaluated by more than one person, the employee should know that as well.
2. Evaluation should be based on concrete, measurable, job-related objectives, and it should focus more on objective issues and less on subjective issues. The skills, behavior, and attitude being evaluated must be job related.

3. The employee should be provided with feedback after the evaluation. This enables the employee to know which areas of job performance need to be improved upon.

4. The evaluator must be fair and not show any favoritism. If an evaluator cannot be objective for any reason in evaluating a particular employee, that evaluator should be replaced (to the extent possible) by someone else.

5. The factors on which the employee will be rated should be prioritized or weighted if appropriate. This will identify and separate the most important factors from the least important. If, however, all aspects of the evaluation are equally important, weighting is not appropriate.

6. The evaluation process should provide employee input and an employee appeal procedure. This is not to say that employees will eventually agree with their evaluation. Opportunity for input gives the employee a chance to provide feedback and possibly explain poor performance.

7. Evaluation should be simple and to the point.

8. Employees should be evaluated by the individual to whom they report directly and with whom they work directly.

Adhering to these basic principles will help prevent employees from reacting with hostility to their performance evaluation. It will also help employees understand that their merits will be recognized and they will not be criticized unfairly.

Why Employees May Perform Poorly

Some of the reasons why employees perform poorly are

- They do not know how to do the job, because they have not been taught the needed skills.
- They think they are performing well, because no one has indicated otherwise.
- They do not know what to do because no one has informed them of their job responsibilities. The manager may have presumed that the employees know or should know what is expected of them.
- The employees do not see their jobs as essential to the organization.
- Some employees are rewarded for not performing: Poor performers are reassigned to easier jobs rather than being held accountable to perform well.
- The employees have a poor attitude toward their job responsibilities and lack enthusiasm for the job.

DISCIPLINARY ACTIONS

Disciplinary actions are an important component of human resources management. They are a contingency measure to be used when other approaches have failed to resolve employee performance problems. One common disciplinary problem in healthcare organizations, in both community and institutional practice, is employee pilferage. (This is discussed in chapter 6.) Other increasingly frequent problems are insubordination, alcoholism, and substance misuse or abuse. One way to deal with these problems is to communicate policies and work rules and make certain that employees understand that these rules are related to job effectiveness. Employees must be informed of the consequences of violating these policies.

A formal procedure for disciplinary action is necessary and employees should be made aware of it. The procedure may begin with an oral reprimand, followed by a written reprimand, then disciplinary suspension without pay, demotion (rarely), and finally discharge.

Oral Reprimand

These are used when an employee fails to maintain certain standards in the workplace. This may involve violating a safety rule, being rude to patients, being chronically late for work, absenteeism, or not following a set procedure. An oral reprimand should be in the form of a corrective action to prevent the problem from recurring. The consequences of the problems recurring should be clearly communicated to the employee. Oral reprimands are for less serious problems and are the lowest level of disciplinary action.

Written Reprimands

These are the next step in the disciplinary process. A written reprimand may not differ from an oral reprimand except that it is in writing and made a part of the employee's record. The disciplined employee should receive a copy of the written reprimand.

Suspension

Disciplinary suspension without pay is next in severity after oral and written reprimands. Usually it lasts for days or weeks. The loss of income associated with this form of disciplinary action makes it severe. Some employers, however, may have difficulty replacing an individual for a few weeks and may skip this stage and discharge the employee instead.

Demotion

This is seldom used as a disciplinary measure. Demotion is used when an employee is no longer willing or able to perform the job. Demotion as a disciplinary action is a source of employee humiliation and loss of motivation. Some employers will ask an employee to resign, or transfer the employee, rather than use demotion.

Discharge

This is the ultimate penalty and is less common than oral and written reprimands. For the employee, it means looking for another job; for the employer, it means the expense of recruiting and training a new employee.

It is important to keep a written record of these disciplinary measures in employee personnel files for protection in possible discrimination lawsuits. Managers must take steps to ensure that the employees' rights are protected at all times, that employees receive copies of all communications, and that they are aware of the meaning of those communications.

Discipline should be directed against a particular unacceptable act by an employee. Its purpose is to maintain compliance with established rules and regulations in the workplace and therefore correct unacceptable conduct. Discipline should not be used to "get even" with an employee. Employees are more likely to accept discipline without resentment when they regard it as fair; unexpected discipline is usually considered unfair.

For discipline to be considered fair, the employees must be informed that

1. A given offense will lead to discipline no matter who they are or what their position in the organization is.
2. A given offense will result in a specific type and duration of disciplinary action.
3. A disciplinary process will be followed for various offenses.
4. Disciplinary actions will be enforced for any and all offenses committed. A disciplinary policy that is not enforced is as good as no policy.

The key to effective disciplinary policy is effective communication within the organization. Effective communication and management will reduce the need for employee disciplinary actions.

GRIEVANCE PROCEDURES

An employee grievance procedure should be established even in the absence of unions. The procedure consists of a formal process for handling complaints. If a healthcare setting is unionized, the procedures and channels are, or should be, established through contract negotiations.

The advantage of a grievance procedure is that it can speed the settlement of small problems. A typical grievance procedure begins with an employee indicating the nature of a grievance to an immediate supervisor, either orally or in writing. At that point, the supervisor attempts to resolve the grievance. If it cannot be solved at the lowest level, it is appealed progressively up the hierarchy. The final step is submitting the grievance to an independent board or committee. In unionized healthcare organizations, arbitration may be carried out through the Federal Mediation and Conciliation Service or the American Arbitration Association. Most grievances, however, are resolved at the lowest level.

An arbitrator makes the final decision—for example, to sustain the organization's action, to reduce the penalty, or to eliminate the penalty. (For more information on arbitration and mediation, see chapter 7.) In small organizations or non-union environments, the grievance committee will make a recommendation to the head of the organization, who will make the final decision. Thus, the grievance procedure serves to protect the employee from unfair treatment. It also serves to maintain consistency and avoid discriminatory discipline in the workplace.

CHAPTER 3 REFERENCES

1. McCormic, E.J.; Jeanneret, P.R.; and Mecham, R.C. "A Study of Job Characteristics and Job Dimensions as Based on the Position Analysis Questionnaire (PAQ)," *Journal of Applied Psychology*, 56, 1972, 347–68.
2. Tornow, W.W., and Pinto, P.R. "The Development of a Managerial Job Tatonomy: A System of Describing, Classifying, and Evaluating Positions." *Journal of Applied Psychology*, 61, 1976, 410–18.
3. Levin, E.L.; Ash, R.A.; and Bennett N. "Explanatory Comparative Study of Four Job Analysis Methods," *Journal of Applied Psychology*, 65, October 1980, 524–35.
4. Ash, R.A., and Levine, E. "A Framework for Evaluating Job Analysis Methods," *Personnel*, 57, November-December 1980, 53–59.
5. Scott, W.D.; Clothier, R.C.; and Spriegel, W.R. *Personnel Management* (New York: McGraw-Hill, 1961).
6. Prien, E.P., and Ronan, W.W. "Job Analysis: A Review of Research Findings," *Personnel*, 24, 1971, 371–96.

7. Lacy, John. "Job Evaluation and EEO," *Employee Relations Law Journal*, 7, #3, 1979, 210–17.

8. Scott, W. D., et al. Op. cit.

9. National Association of Chain Drug Stores (NACDS) *Executive Newsletter*, July 16, 1973.

10. Commerce Clearing House *Employment Practices Guide*, August 3, 1972, 1193.

11. Howell, M.L. "Complying With the Fair Credit Reporting Act," *The Personnel Administrator*, 17, January-February 1972, 10–12.

12. Maanen, John Van. "Breaking In: Socialization to Work," in Robert Dubin, ed., *Handbook of Work, Organization and Society* (Chicago: Rand McNally Publishing Company, 1976).

13. Gomersall, Earl R., and Myers, Scott M. "Break Through in On-the-Job Training," *Harvard Business Review*, July-August 1966, 62–71.

14. Marion, B.W. and Trieb, S.E. "Job Orientation: A Factor in Employee Performance and Turnover," *Personnel Journal*, October 1969, 779–804.

15. Weitz, J. "Job Expectancy: An Important Factor in Labor Turnover," *Personnel Journal*, May 1972, 360–363.

16. Scott, R.D. "Job Expectancy and Survival," *Journal of Applied Psychology*, 40, 1956, 245–247.

17. Patton, J.A., and Littlefield, C.A. *Job Evaluation* (Homewood, IL: Richard D. Irwin, 1957).

18. Baggaley, A.R. "A Scheme for Classifying Rating Methods," *Personnel Psychology*, 27, 1974, 139–44.

19. Smith, P.C., and Kendall, L.M., "Retranslating of Expectations: An Approach to the Construction of Ambiguous Anchors for Rating Scales," *Journal of Applied Psychology*, 47, 1973, 149–55.

20. Campbell, J.P.; Dunnettle, M.D.; Arvey, R.D.; and Helllervik, L.V. "The Development and Evaluation of Behaviorally Based Rating Scales," *Journal of Applied Psychology*, 57, 1973, 15–22.

21. Schwab, D.P., Heneman, H.C., and DeCotis, T.A. "Behaviorally Based Rating Scales: A Review of the Literature," *Personnel Psychology*, 28, 1975, 549–62.

Group Dynamics 4

Cohesiveness and teamwork are very important in managing any health-care facility work group. A work group consists of two or more individuals who interdependently accomplish the goals and objectives set by the organization. The work group interacts and works together. Work groups with good relationships also help in satisfying employees need for growth and meeting organizational goals.

JOB SATISFACTION

Job satisfaction comprises an individual's reaction to, attitude toward, and perceptions of work. Job satisfaction is related to two perceptions held by the employee: what the work is and what the work should be.[1] If an employee believes that the job is what it should be, the employee will be satisfied. However, if the employee's perception of what the job should be exceeds what it is, the employee may become dissatisfied.

Job satisfaction consists of the affective reactions of a person to a combination of different aspects, or facets, of responsibility in the work environment. It consists of many complex sets of variables.

Factors Influencing Job Satisfaction

Some of the factors that influence job satisfaction will be discussed under three general categories. The three major sources of job satisfaction or dissatisfaction among employees are

1. Organizational policy and procedures.
2. Other employees.
3. The work itself.

Organizational Policy and Procedures

This category includes income and fringe benefits, social interaction at work, advancement and promotions, and the work schedule.

Income and Fringe Benefits

Money can be a source of job satisfaction or dissatisfaction. The degree of its influence varies from one individual to another. The influence of money as a source of job dissatisfaction has been found with individuals at higher occupational levels.[2] When an employee feels underpaid compared with other employees in the same job category, this leads to dissatisfaction. This is one reason an employee may leave to work for another employer in the same position or a similar one. If the employee remains with the employer but does not receive a pay increase, the employee may reduce job performance to a level that the employee thinks matches the pay. The underpaid employee may also steal from the employer, justifying the theft as a means of making up the difference between what the employee is paid and what the employee thinks the work is worth.

Another source of employee job satisfaction or dissatisfaction is fringe benefits—such things as being able to get time off to attend to personal matters, product or service discounts provided by the employer, a health insurance program, paid vacation, sick leave, and pension plans. The more fringe benefits an employee gets, the more satisfied the employee is likely to be, especially if the fringe benefits are those the employee perceives to be important and needed.

Social Interaction at Work

This is one of the major sources of employee satisfaction or dissatisfaction in the work environment. Social interaction at work gives employees a sense of belonging. As a result, many individuals, including retirees, prefer to continue working even when they do not need the money.[3] Individuals with high social needs may prefer to work in an environment where this need is fulfilled even if the pay is less than they could earn elsewhere. If these people work in isolation, they are more likely to be dissatisfied with their jobs. The degree of social interaction needed in a healthcare work environment will differ from one setting to another, but it serves three major functions:

1. Emotional support for the employees as they perform their work.
2. Satisfaction of complex social needs.
3. Assistance in meeting goals.

Other employees, by providing emotional support, can help an individual employee define the basis of ethical behavior and identify desirable and undesirable behavior in the work environment. Other people, with stronger self-identification or a stronger conscience, will be more likely to stand against a group or initiate action on their own without seeking group support.

When an employee is going through difficult emotional times, such as serious illness or a death in the family, emotional support from other employees helps the person cope.

Satisfaction of complex social needs is another function served by employee social interaction. Social interaction at work gives an employee a sense of affiliation, a sense of belonging. The basis of affiliation could be simple enjoyment of other people's company or the more complex need for group affirmation of an individuals' self-concept. Employees with no opportunity for social interaction are more likely to be dissatisfied with their work, which may result in poor performance, high turnover, and a higher rate of absenteeism compared with employees who interact.

Fellow employees do more than provide emotional support and satisfy social needs, however, they also assist each other in meeting the goals of the organization they work for. Employees can help each other solve problems. For example, a new technician who is unsure of a procedure will be more likely to ask a more experienced employee for help than to ask the supervisor or, worse still, risk harming the patient with an inappropriate procedure. Therefore, employee interaction is not only desirable but should be encouraged in healthcare organizations. Occasional social events, such as office parties, are a way of encouraging social interaction between the employer and the employees, and among employees.

Advancement and Promotions

Dissatisfaction among professionals is often attributed to the lack of opportunity for advancement and self-actualization.[4,5] An employee's advancement and promotion usually mean more responsibilities, which may require new skills.

Some individuals seek promotion for job satisfaction and not necessarily for increased income. Others seek promotion primarily to increase income. It is therefore important to determine why an individual is seeking promotion, since it may be possible to satisfy the employee's need without promotion to another position. For example, an employee may be satisfied with a pay raise or some other form of recognition without promotion.

The Work Schedule

This is another source of job satisfaction or dissatisfaction among employees. Work schedules that continuously infringe on employees' leisure or personal time create job dissatisfaction. Requiring employees to work overtime when this disrupts family responsibilities creates problems. Even during work hours, employees sometimes need to attend to family or personal obligations outside work. The more flexible a work schedule is in allowing employees to attend to occasional personal matters, the more satisfied employees are likely to be.

Other Employees

Although social interaction in the work environment is important and a source of job satisfaction, other employees can also be a source of satisfaction or dissatisfaction. Obnoxious, lazy, and uncooperative employees are a source of job dissatisfaction for their fellow employees. When an employee does not perform adequately and that inadequacy is allowed to continue, other employees will become dissatisfied.

Supervision can also be a factor in job satisfaction. A supervisor's attitude, expectations, supervision style, and relationship with other employees can be a source of high or low employee morale. Employees may be more satisfied when their supervisor is fair to everyone and, to some extent, employee oriented rather than extremely task oriented.

Enthusiastic employees also can create an enthusiastic work environment. On the other hand, slow, sluggish, and dull employees create a dull and possibly depressing workplace, which can be a source of job dissatisfaction to other employees.

The Work Itself

Some healthcare professionals, such as some pharmacists, nurses, and those in allied health professions, depend on the physician to initiate a work order for them to carry on their responsibilities. For such healthcare professionals[6] the partial lack of control over their profession and activities—having to depend on another profession to initiate an order, for example—has been indicated as a source of considerable dissatisfaction, anxiety, and frustration, especially where there is a strained relationship between the professionals.

Working conditions such as safety in the workplace, room temperature, space, and lighting will also affect job satisfaction and may lead to high employee turnover.[7] The issue of safety is one that should be of concern not only to the employees but also to the employer. It is the employer's responsibility to provide a safe work environment for employees and patients. If an employee is injured or killed in a workplace as a result of unsafe conditions, the employer may be liable for damages. The Occupational Safety and Health Act (OSHA) requires safe and healthful working conditions. The legislation makes management responsible for identifying safety hazards and protecting employees from them. The law provides fines and penalties for violations, and employees who file work safety charges are protected under the law from retaliation. The law also grants the right to be informed of their exposure to all toxic or hazardous materials, and to observe federal inspections and organizational control procedures. A safety manual for employees should be prepared and enforced in compliance with applicable laws.

Although job repetition and monotony may cause job dissatisfaction because the work is not challenging, some individuals are less susceptible to monotony and boredom. It is the responsibility of the supervisor to make sure that monotonous jobs are assigned to individuals who are less susceptible to becoming bored and therefore dissatisfied. Otherwise jobs should be varied to avoid boredom.

If an employee is mismatched with a job, it becomes a source of dissatisfaction. Mismatching occurs when an employee is either overly qualified or not sufficiently qualified for a job. An overqualified employee is unable to use all his or her skills, and may become frustrated and dissatisfied. Such employees may leave when they find another job opportunity more suited to their qualifications. If an employee is not qualified for a job, this creates tension because of the employee's inability to perform the required tasks. Employers should avoid assigning employees to tasks for which they are not qualified, because they may cause serious harm to themselves, to others, or to patients. Other employees will notice the inadequacies of the mismatched employee, and this can be embarrassing for that employee and a source of resentment from those who have to help the mismatched employee do the job correctly.

The pressure to produce, such as to fill a certain number of prescriptions, or to see a certain number of patients a day, builds up tension and may result in job dissatisfaction as well as increased errors. Work requiring a short completion time irritates employees when they also have to deal with distractions that are not necessarily related to the task at hand. This usually occurs when an organization is understaffed. For example, a pharmacist might be expected to fill a high volume of prescriptions, counsel patients, answer the phones, and run the cash register.

Consequences of Job Dissatisfaction

Job dissatisfaction is undesirable because of its negative consequences. Some of these include:

- Job stress, with possible serious health implications.
- Decreased productivity and poor work quality.
- Low morale.
- High employee turnover.
- A gloomy work environment.

Improving Job Satisfaction

Job satisfaction can be improved by dealing with the sources and reasons for the dissatisfaction. This can be achieved by making organizational policy and procedures a source of job satisfaction, handling of other employees issues effectively, and making the work itself a source of job satisfaction.

Ways of Making Organizational Policy and Procedures a Source of Job Satisfaction

- Provide employees with adequate job descriptions and expectations.
- Provide a policy and procedures manual to employees.
- Provide adequate wages and fringe benefits commensurate with the job.
- Provide an environment for social interaction.
- Develop an appropriate work schedule that allows some flexibility for employees to attend to personal matters.
- Provide opportunities for promotion and advancement.
- Provide appropriate mechanisms for employee evaluation and feedback.
- Listen to employee grievances.
- Establish clear lines of authority in the work environment.

Ways of Effectively Handling Other Employees Issues to Improve Job Satisfaction

- Develop an appropriate leadership style in the work environment.
- Reduce personality problems among employees.
- Allow proper social interaction in the workplace.

Ways of Making Work Itself a Source of Job Satisfaction

- Improve working conditions.
- Provide variety in the job, where possible, to avoid boredom.
- Get the right person for the right job. Be sure employee and employer job expectations are similar.
- Provide adequate staffing in the healthcare setting.

As indicated earlier, job dissatisfaction can be caused by a lack of control over the hours of work and a lack of flexibility in the working hours to meet personal needs. To deal with this problem, various types of flexible work scheduling have been implemented in various work environments to improve job satisfaction and employee relations. These more flexible, non-traditional types of work scheduling include

- The four-day work week.
- Use of flex-time.
- Job sharing.

These will be discussed in detail in the following section to help you determine whether any or all of them could be useful in your healthcare setting.

The Four-Day Work Week

This scheduling technique allows employees to have more time off from work while still working full time. The four-day or compressed work week usually means scheduling 10 hours a day for four days, allowing the employee to have three days off each week. Which four days an employee works depend on organizational needs. Some healthcare settings, such as clinics, are open six days a week and some are open 24 hours a day.[8,9,10] In some instances, fewer than 40 hours per week are worked for 40 hours pay. Some organizations use the four-day work week as a recruiting tool.[11] When this form of work week fails, it can sometimes be attributed to inadequate planning and poor management. Before changing to a four-day work week, an organization should consider its goals and evaluate the employees' attitude toward the revised schedule. Even if the supervisor or manager feels that it is a workable and excellent idea, it should not be instituted if the employees do not want it. If the employees do want a four-day work week, they should be involved in the planning to make it more effective. The four-day work week has some advantages as well as disadvantages, which are identified below.

Advantages of the Four-Day Work Week

- Improved morale and productivity.
- Decreased absenteeism, since employees have more time off to take care of personal matters.
- Increased employee leisure time.
- Its use as a recruitment tool.
- A possible reduction of incentive for employees to unionize.
- Improved job satisfaction.

Disadvantages of the Four-Day Work Week

- Working 10 hours a day rather than the traditional 8 may increase employee fatigue and result in decreased quality of work.
- It may lead to employee pressure for a 36-hour week for 40 hours pay.
- It may not be suitable for some employees. This disadvantage can be avoided if the four-day week is made available only to those who want it.
- It may not be suitable in some work settings, such as those with very few employees, those that are open only on weekdays from 8:00 in the morning to 5:00 in the afternoon, or where each employee provides a specialized, specific service that other employees cannot provide in that employee's absence.

Flex-Time

Another technique to increase work schedule flexibility and allow employees more time to attend to personal matters is flex-time. Under flex-time, employees have more flexibility in the work schedule.[12,13,14] It requires only that employees be present for a certain period in the morning or afternoon, with the remaining work hours to be completed within a specified time at the employee's discretion. Flex-time can be applied to both full-time and part-time employees.

Under daily flex-time, the employee works the full eight hours but chooses starting and ending times within the organization's hours of operation. Under weekly flex-time, employees complete a 40-hour work week but may work more hours in one day and less in another. Before instituting weekly flex-time for employees who are paid by the hour, it is prudent to check current wage-hour laws to avoid paying overtime in a week when an employee works more than 40 hours. In some organizations using flex-time, the total hours are calculated on a biweekly or monthly basis rather than weekly. In any of these flex-time arrangements, lunch times may be fixed or flexible. Flex-time has advantages as well as disadvantages. Some of these are outlined below.

Advantages of Flex-time

- Flex-time recognizes that people differ in their physiological cycles and mental states during the day. It allows employees to adjust their working hours to when they are more likely to be most productive.
- Flex-time treats employees as responsible adults and gives them ownership of their work schedule.
- Flex-time decreases employee tardiness, turnover, and absenteeism.
- Flex-time gives employees an opportunity to adjust their work schedules to fit their lifestyles; it especially benefits employees who have to drop off and pick up their children from day care centers, babysitters, or school.
- Used effectively, flex-time can increase job satisfaction.
- Flex-time can decrease the tension of getting to work every day by a certain time.
- Employees can have more leisure time if they desire it.
- Flex-time increases production, morale and employee performance.
- Flex-time reduces requests by employees for personal time off.

Disadvantages of Flex-time

- Flex-time can cause supervision problems, especially if it is not well organized and monitored.
- Flex-time may create problems in keeping records of hours worked if a time-clock is not used.
- Flex-time may conflict with wage laws, especially overtime pay of hourly employees. However, this problem may be resolved by using a weekly system and calculating the hours worked on a weekly basis, requiring hourly wage employees not to exceed 40 hours in any week. It is prudent to make sure the law will not require employers to pay overtime.

- Flex-time is difficult to implement in work settings with only one employee, or organizations that are in operation for eight hours or less a day. In such settings, job sharing may work better.

Job Sharing

In this form of work scheduling, two part-time employees fill a position that otherwise would be held by one full-time employee. The work is split between employees working at two different times. Flex-time can be implemented along with job-sharing if the employees desire it. Some of the advantages and disadvantages of job sharing are identified below.[15]

Advantages of Job Sharing

- It is excellent for individuals who want to work part-time, such as students or individuals who have more than one job.
- The employer saves money on fringe benefits if they are available only to full-time employees.
- Employees have more time off to attend to personal matters, resulting in fewer requests for time off.
- Job sharing decreases absenteeism and turnover.
- It improves job satisfaction.

Disadvantages of Job Sharing

- It increases recruitment, training, and orientation costs, since the organization has to train two employees for one full-time position.
- There is a risk of personality conflict between the employees sharing a position.
- Part-time employees often do not get the fringe benefits, such as paid vacation, available to full-time employees.

EMPLOYEE MOTIVATION

A necessary part of personnel management involves learning and implementing work conditions in which people can be stimulated or motivated to improve job performance. Healthcare organization supervisors and managers who want to motivate employees will increase their chances of doing so when they understand employees work-related needs. Employee motivation in general and motivating employees in a healthcare organization to perform their best are complex issues.

Motivation can be explained as individual needs or desires that cause or impel a person to act. Employees' needs or drives, the goals toward which their behavior is directed, and the rewards they receive for achieving these goals all affect motivation. What motivates one employee may not motivate another or may not motivate the same employee in a different situation.

THEORIES OF EMPLOYEE MOTIVATION

Numerous needs have been identified and studied, resulting in several theories of motivation. However, there are a few basic categories of needs that are generally accepted as being able to motivate employees.

Some of the basic motivation theories are the following:

- The hierarchy-of-needs-theory.
- The two-factor theory.
- Expectancy theory.
- Reinforcement theory.
- Goal-setting theory.

The Hierarchy-of-Needs Theory

Maslow's hierarchy-of-needs theory has gained wide acceptance as a theory of employee motivation. According to Maslow, there are five distinct hierarchical needs: physiological, safety, love or sense of belonging, esteem, and self-actualization,[16,17] (see figure 13).

Physiological needs are at the bottom of the hierarchy, while self-actualization needs are at the top. This does not mean that self-actualization is more important than physiological needs. What motivates an employee is a function of that employee's pattern of need satisfaction in the hierarchy. A person may start out aspiring to satisfy esteem needs but be driven to satisfy lower needs if those become unsatisfied.

Physiological Needs

These are the most basic needs in the hierarchy. They include but are not limited to the need for food, water, air, shelter, and clothing, which are all needed to maintain life. As long as these needs are unsatisfied, they remain strong motivators, and new and higher needs are unlikely to emerge. An employee who desperately needs a job to pay for essential living expenses is often motivated to perform well because that individual's livelihood depends on the job. To an individual without food, the need for food is a

Figure 13. *Illustration of Maslow's Hierarchy-of-Needs Theory*

HIGHEST NEED	SELF-ACTUALIZATION
	ESTEEM NEEDS
	LOVE NEEDS
	SAFETY NEEDS
LOWEST NEED	PHYSIOLOGICAL NEEDS

potent motivator. However, as physiological needs are met—at least at a minimum level—new and higher needs emerge to motivate behavior.

Safety Needs

The need for security and safety includes being free from harm in the physical work environment. Safety needs occupy the next level in the hierarchy, and become a major motivator after the physiological needs are satisfied. Safety needs also include being free from fear and anxiety, and having job security. Efforts to satisfy safety needs resulted in the development and growth of unions. Some unions were instrumental in the development of safe work environments, pension plans, various health insurance policies, and seniority systems to govern employee layoffs. An employee whose physiological needs have been met will now seek to protect the source that meets those needs.

According to the hierarchy-of-needs theory, as lower level needs are relatively satisfied, they become less important in directly motivating an employee's behavior. Thus, gratified and met needs in a sense disappear as a motivator, and the next level of unsatisfied needs becomes an important employee motivator.

Love Needs

Individuals generally have strong needs to interact and associate with other people. This category includes the need to belong, be loved, socialize, be socially satisfied, and be accepted in the work environment. Individuals generally desire affectionate, nonhostile relationships with other people. In the healthcare setting, a friendly working relationship among employees is a major source of satisfying the love need and should be encouraged. It also gives employees a sense of belonging in the organization. Social gatherings in the work environment are often held to satisfy employee love needs and improve morale. Such activities do not have to be elaborate. They can occur during the lunch break. Having punch and cake to celebrate an employee's birthday, to welcome an employee back to work after a special absence, or to mark an employee's retirement, helps meet employee needs for love. For these occasions to be productive rather than a source of employee dissatisfaction, a fair amount of consistency must be maintained and each employee given adequate opportunity to participate.

When social or love needs are relatively satisfied, the next hierarchy of need—the desire for esteem—tends to emerge as a motivator.

Esteem Needs

This involves the desire to be respected by others (esteem from others) and to be respected by oneself (self-esteem). An employee's job plays a prominent role in determining self-esteem and the esteem received from others. Having a job is not necessarily a guarantee of deriving esteem from it. However, the organization with which an employee is affiliated is a possible source of self-esteem. The need for esteem from others includes the need for recognition, appreciation, status, prestige, respect, and dignity. Self-esteem or self-respect, on the other hand, includes feelings of competence, autonomy, confidence, and achievement. The esteem needs may be an outgrowth of the love needs, since there seems to be an overlap between the need for belonging and that for affection. One of the esteem needs that has been researched extensively is the need for achievement.[18]

The achievement need displays itself in an individual as an intense concern with setting moderately risky and difficulty goals, working to achieve the goals, and seeking feedback and recognition for success. This need can be satisfied by providing employees with an opportunity to excel through job enrichment. Job enrichment involves expanding jobs both vertically and horizontally, identifying varied tasks and scheduling a time span over which the individual should produce results. It does not mean overloading an employee with added responsibilities. Job enrichment appropriately implemented gives an employee a sense of accomplishment, pride, and respect as the employee accomplishes the tasks.

Esteem needs can also be achieved through employee recognition when an employee makes an outstanding contribution in the workplace. This recognition can take various forms. Examples include awards for employee of the year or month, awards to recognize achievement, salary or wage increases and promotion. Employee-of-the-month recognition is more appropriate in very large organizations. Recognition by an employer or supervisor may be formal or informal. Formal recognition awards may be made during an elaborate social event such as a banquet, which might be completely funded by the employer.

Another means of satisfying esteem needs is for the employer to provide employees with physical manifestations of status differences. In large organizations this may include larger office space, a large equipment laboratory, a name plate on the door or desk, an individual office with a scenic view, an office with a window, an office with more sophisticated equipment, or a special parking space.

Self-actualization or Self-fulfillment

According to the hierarchy-of-needs theory, the peak of psychological development is self-actualization. Self-actualization is the desire to reach one's full, unique potential and become what one is most capable of becoming. An active need for employee self-fulfillment may pose a more subtle and complex motivation challenge to healthcare supervisors and managers than that posed by any of the lower needs. The need for self-fulfillment or self-actualization is distinctive in that it does not seem to terminate in satisfaction,[19] rather, it seems to remain insatiable and important. However, the workplace should be conducive to employees' striving to reach their full potential.

How much each of the needs in the hierarchy will motivate an employee depends very much on the individual. Therefore, the supervisor should consider individual differences. One employee's esteem need may be satisfied by a salary increase, while another employee may prefer an award, a large private office or a promotion, even if it is not associated with an appreciable salary increase.

The Two-Factor Theory

Another motivational theory is the two-factor theory. Herzberg developed a motivation-hygiene theory based on satisfaction and dissatisfaction expressed by employees through an in-depth research interview.[20] Herzberg called those factors that produce job satisfaction motivators, and those that do not produce job satisfaction hygiene factors.

Motivators

These factors, when present, increase job satisfaction and motivate employees to perform better, but when absent they do not lead to dissatisfaction. Herzberg identified the following as motivators:

1. Achievement.
2. Recognition for achievement.
3. Work itself.
4. Responsibility.
5. Advancement.

According to Herzberg, these motivate employees to a high level of performance.

Hygiene Factors

These prevent dissatisfaction, but do not result in positive motivation or satisfaction. However, the absence of hygiene factors often leads to job dissatisfaction. Hygiene factors, according to Herzberg's theory, include

1. Organizational policy and administration in the workplace.
2. Supervisor's management style.
3. Salary.
4. Interpersonal relations.
5. Working conditions.

Hygiene factors may represent an individual's need to avoid discomfort and pain.

Like other motivational theories, the motivator-hygiene theory, also referred to as the two-factor theory, has stimulated some research and criticism.[21] Most of the criticism was related to the research methodology and the theory's disregard for the issue of whether a factor can cause job satisfaction for one person and dissatisfaction for another in the same workplace. A highly structured work environment may satisfy one employee and dissatisfy another. A certain supervision style may encourage one employee to strive yet be suffocating for another.

Expectancy Theory

Vroom's expectancy theory argues that the motivational force to perform is a function of employee anticipation of a valued future outcome. Its central

Figure 14. *Illustration of Expectancy Theory in Relation to Employee Motivation*

---

(1) Need for reward

(2) Belief that performance is necessary to get reward

(3) Performance can be achieved. (Benefits outweigh barriers to performance)

Reward becomes a motivator.

---

idea is that people behave as they do because they perceive that the behavior will lead to a desired reward. Vroom defined an expectancy as a momentary belief concerning the likelihood that a particular performance will be followed by an outcome.[22] Expectancies thus serve as guidelines by which an individual can plan to fulfill personal needs. The expectancy theory emphasizes an individual's perception as being more important in motivating employees than the perception of the supervisor. Reward will, therefore, motivate employees when they have a need for the reward and also believe that performance is necessary and possible to get the reward.

Expectancy theory stresses that (1) the individual must believe that reasonable efforts toward performance can lead to a successful performance; (2) the situation is one in which it is possible to perform; and (3) performance will lead to a worthy reward (see figure 14).

Thus, for a reward to be a motivator, the employee must need the reward. If the employee has not perceived the need for the potential reward, that reward will not be a motivator for that employee. If an employee does not need the reward or feels that it is worthless, the employee will not perform. In addition to needing the reward, the employee must also believe that performance is necessary to get the reward. If employees are rewarded without the required performance, that reward ceases to be a motivator; the employee fails to see performance as necessary to receive the reward. Also, it is necessary for the employee to believe that performance is possible. If an employer requires a very difficult or impossible task for an employee to receive the reward, often the employee will decide not to perform and to forgo the reward. The key to performance is the employee's perception of the need for the reward, the necessity of performance to get rewarded, and the possibility of performance or achieving the desired goal. What the employer or supervisor thinks is not important in motivating performance.

Reinforcement Theory

This theory emphasizes that employee behavior and motivation are contingent upon reinforcement. The theory is based on the Law of Effect.[23] Behavior that results in the satisfaction of employee needs tends to reoccur, while behavior that leads to dissatisfaction tends not be repeated. Thus, performance is a function of what behavior gets rewarded by the employer.

The process of influencing behavior through reinforcement can be achieved through operant conditioning and behavior modification.[24] The shorter the time interval between the behavior and the reinforcement, the more likely the behavior will be influenced to continue. Therefore, it is better to reward an employee for a job well done soon after the performance.

The greater the reward that employees perceive they will receive for performing, the more likely they will strive to perform in the accepted manner so as to receive the reward. Tasks or performance requiring more effort are less often performed than those requiring less effort. Also, the more complex the required task, the more it will be avoided. Therefore, it is better to break down difficult tasks into several simple tasks to improve the frequency and quality of employee performance.

Goal-Setting Theory

This theory emphasizes that having specific goals for employees increases performance and therefore motivates employees.[25,26] Goal-setting theory is similar to Management by Objective (MBO) in that it focuses on employees' setting goals within a framework provided by the supervisor to meet the overall goals of the organization.[27] In using goal-setting theory to motivate employees, it is important to note the following:

1. Each goal must be specific and clear to the employee.
2. There must be a reasonable time limit for the achievement of each goal.
3. Each goal must be measurable, quantitatively or qualitatively.
4. Each goal must be achievable within the allocated timeframe.
5. Intermediate goals may be necessary to achieve overall goals.
6. Goals may be modified, changed, or abandoned when appropriate.

7. Employees must understand the role of thier goals in successfully achieving the overall goal of the organization.

(Management by Objective was discussed in chapter 2. Refer to that chapter for more information.)

Motivation and Management

The more a supervisor can tie an employee's task performance to increasing the employee's job satisfaction, the higher the probability that the employee's efforts will be committed to organizational purposes. Although motives and needs may be invisible, their presence can be inferred from behavior. Supervisors can often infer what employees want from what they say and do. It is best when in doubt to discuss motives and needs with the employee. Effective communication is very important in determining what motivates a particular employee and what does not.

Individuals differ in their relative needs and how intensely those needs are likely to motivate them. While some individuals remain strongly influenced by certain needs, others are not necessarily influenced by the same ones. It is the responsibility of those in supervisory roles to determine which needs strongly motivate their employees.

CONFLICT IN THE WORKPLACE

Conflict occurs when there is a clash between opposing views. Conflicts can be competitive or disruptive. Competitive conflicts result when employees seek limited resources. Anger during conflicts causes disruption, such that employees may abandon pursuit of organizational goals and engage in irrational acts of aggression.

Types of Conflict

Intrapersonal Conflict

This type of conflict exists within an individual as a result of having various needs. A healthcare professional may seek to start a successful, private, independent professional practice in a community setting. The individual may succeed but then become dissatisfied by the lack of time left to attend to personal and family matters or the restrictions imposed by third parties such as managed care organizations and insurance companies in the reimbursement of healthcare services provided to patients.

Interpersonal Conflict

Interpersonal conflict can be a group versus an individual or one individual versus another. Conflict may occur when an employee tries to satisfy a love need (the need to belong) through other employees if the colleagues demand an unacceptable or difficult behavior from the individual as a condition of acceptance. A group-versus-individual conflict can occur when an individual wants to promote personal interests at the expense of other employees, or by breaking the group's norms or rules. Conflict may also occur when an individual highly distinguishes himself or herself and other employees feel threatened by that person's achievement.

Reasons for Conflict

A conflict of one individual versus another occurs as individuals compete for promotion, limited resources, power, status, prestige, etc. Conflict among employees can also occur as a result of the following:[28,29]

1. Poor communication, which results in misunderstanding and may cause conflict. For example, a well-meaning suggestion from one employee to another on how to improve job performance may be misunderstood or resisted because the suggestion is seen as one employee telling the other what to do.
2. Conflict of interest—this occurs where the goals of the organization compete with the personal goals of the employee. Conflict of interest may also occur when an employee works for an employer's competitor.
3. Unclear lines of authority—these become a problem because the employee appears to have several supervisors at the same time, and the employee is unclear whom to report to.
4. A need for consensus—if attempts to reach consensus are seen as forcing agreement, they may result in conflict.
5. Unclear job description and employee roles—these create conflict because the employee is unsure of what the job responsibilities are.
6. Territorial encroachment—this results in conflict because an employee perceives a particular work area as personal territory. When another employee gets into that area, that is seen as encroaching. For example, if a lab is seen and referred to as Dr. Doe's lab, that creates an environment for territorial encroachment, because the lab is perceived by employees as belonging to Dr. Doe, not to the healthcare organization.

7. Interaction patterns—the way individual employees interact at work may cause conflict. This can create pockets of people who cling together against other employees who are not part of their group.
8. Conflicting loyalties—these are similar to conflict of interest. In this instance the employees have divided loyalty and therefore are not completely loyal to their employer.
9. Separation of knowledge and authority—If employees' knowledge, skills, education, and experience have no bearing on their level of authority—for example, if a supervisor is not knowledgeable about the work accomplished by subordinates—there is a high probability of conflict in the workplace.
10. Incompatible styles—when management style is contrary to employee needs, conflict is likely to occur. For example, a supervisor's leadership style that requires employee initiative and some autonomy may conflict with an employee's desire for constant guidance, direction, and supervision.
11. Change versus stability—change causes conflict where the change is perceived by the employees as a threat to their way of doing things rather than as an opportunity for improvement. The supervisor may hear comments like "We have always done it this way," "No one has complained about this before, so why change now?" or "If it is not broken, why fix it?"
12. Work flow—this becomes a source of conflict where some employees are loaded with work while others have little or nothing to do, especially if the workload could easily be better allocated.

Conflict Resolution

Our political system uses the one-person, one-vote approach to problem solving. Decisions are based on which solution receives majority acceptance, even though opposition is present and differences remain unresolved. This creates winners (the majority) and losers (the minorities). Legal methods of conflict resolution, such as use of the court system, apply only when the question involves the law and other means have been unsatisfactory in resolving the problem or reaching a decision. In formal organizations, hierarchy can permit the resolution of differences. It can be done through the legitimate power resulting from an individual's position in the organization. The individual higher up imposes a decision on those below. This method does not provide a sound and sufficient basis for true problem solving[30] in the work environment.

Research has indicated that group problem solving and decision making produce higher acceptance of the decision and a higher probability that the decision will be executed efficiently in the work environment. Most healthcare organizations, especially larger ones, have a diversified workforce including professional, semiprofessional, skilled, and technical employees. Such diversity of employees in a healthcare organization makes the work environment prone to constant confrontation. Managers face the challenge of resolving tension, conflict, and friction arising from misinformation, misunderstandings, and disagreements. In resolving disruptive interpersonal and interdepartmental conflicts, it is essential that the supervisor develop the ability to resolve conflicts if organizational goals are to be adequately met.

Various strategies exist for effectively handling conflicts in the workplace.[31,32,33,34,35,36] Some basic strategies for dealing with conflict include the following:

1. The win-lose strategy
2. The lose-lose strategy
3. The win-win strategy
4. Other strategies:
   - Withdrawing
   - Smoothing
   - Compromising
   - Forcing
   - Confronting

The Win-Lose Strategy

The win-lose method of conflict resolution creates winners and losers, often similar to the results achieved through majority vote. An individual in a supervisory role who sees conflict as a personal threat may use the win-lose approach, using supervisory authority to impose a decision on employees. The supervisor feels like a winner, while the employees (who may not be in a position to object) become losers. This approach to conflict resolution gives the supervisor a sense of being in control in negotiations with employees, causing one-way communication patterns. Employees working with such an individual often feel intense frustration if they are unable to develop strategies for coping with this win-lose style. The employees may therefore feel that no matter what they do, the supervisor will eventually impose a decision on them to get his or her own way. The employees in this instance may communicate to the supervisor only what the supervisor wants to hear. This becomes a mechanism or strategy for the employees to avoid direct confrontation with the supervisor. In such a situation the healthcare organization loses, because energy that would have been used in constructive problem solving and conflict resolution is wasted either in confrontation or in avoiding confrontation between the supervisor and employees. The win–lose method creates a we-versus-them orientation in problem solving and should be avoided, because it polarizes those involved in a conflict situation.

The Lose-Lose Strategy

The lose–lose strategy in conflict resolution results from compromise such that individuals in the conflict do not achieve all they wanted. No one emerges as a winner. The individuals get only some of what they required. While compromise may sometimes be necessary, it is not the best means of conflict resolution. The lose–lose method is based on the assumption that half a loaf is better than none and that avoidance of conflict is preferable to personal confrontation.[37] This strategy is often used when employees have a specific solution to a problem but feel that those in charge would not accept it. In such a situation, the employees and the supervisor arrive at the best solution under the circumstances, compromising to avoid offending either party.

In both the win–lose and lose–lose strategies, there is a clear distinction between the needs of the parties and the solutions that would be acceptable to each. Their attitude is "I versus you" rather than "we versus the problem," solving the problem together in the best interest of the organization. In the lose–lose strategy, the individual personalities, rather than ways in which the problem can be approached and resolved, often become the main issue. Thus, lose–lose conflict resolution revolves around personal perspectives rather than the organizational perspective. The win–lose and lose–lose methods of conflict resolution are ineffective in dealing with problems that require solutions of high quality and high acceptance. Whether a defined solution satisfactorily resolves a given conflict for those involved will be determined by the commitment everyone involved feels toward the solution.

The Win-Win Strategy

The win–win strategy is another method of dealing with conflict. It not only focuses on consensus but requires individuals to express their needs and ideas. It seeks to produce solutions acceptable to all individuals. For a win-win solution to be achieved, all parties must be open and honest about facts, opinions, and feelings. As much as is feasible, all facts regarding the conflict should be revealed. It is difficult to solve a conflict without information. When an individual is evasive concerning the reasons for strongly advocating a position, distrust tends to arise, which interferes with reaching a solution acceptable to all. The win-win approach is based on the conviction that serious problems are best solved using well-defined, process-oriented decision-making methods. A problem-solving process that is defined, agreed to by those involved in the conflict, and implemented as agreed increases the probability of achieving effective conflict resolution. For effective conflict resolution, defensiveness, anxiety, and hostility must be diminished during the process so that creative solutions can emerge. To achieve a win-win solution in conflict resolution, supervisors should adopt and practice a problem-solving style of approaching and managing conflict that allows open participation and commitment to a solution that is acceptable to all.

There are other strategies and approaches that can be used in conflict situations. Some of these approaches may overlap, facilitate, or complement the win-lose, lose-lose, or win-win strategies. These approaches may also be used temporarily when appropriate during the process of problem solving with the eventual goal of achieving a win-win solution. These approaches include the following.

Other Strategies

1. Withdrawing
2. Smoothing
3. Compromising
4. Forcing
5. Confronting[38]

Withdrawing

In withdrawing from a conflict in order to resolve it, action is initiated only on pressing issues, and only when it is absolutely necessary. When a supervisor cannot withdraw, another tack is maintaining strict neutrality by not giving any personal opinion.[39] The problem with this is that the conflict remains unresolved. Withdrawal or neutrality is like trying to sweep conflict under the rug and hoping that it will go away. Withdrawing may therefore be seen as inaction.

Smoothing

The individual who smooths conflicts often has a low tolerance for disagreements and expression of negative emotions. The smoother emphasizes the positive, saying, "Look on the bright side, it can't be all that bad." This does not necessarily result in an effective working environment. Employees can become frustrated because issues are not confronted, and the supervisor is generally too nice a person to deal with them effectively. Since issues are not addressed, there is no opportunity for a win-win solution. It is possible, however, to use smoothing within a win-win strategy. This is not merely smoothing, but a means to achieve a win-win solution.

Compromising

The compromise approach is similar to the lose-lose method of conflict resolution, in that the supervisor decides on a position in which all individuals feel relatively comfortable. If confronted with a serious disagreement, the supervisor seeking a compromise may suggest some mechanism (such as voting) for finding a workable solution rather than working out the disagreement to find the best solution.[40] The basic limitation of a compromise approach is related to the intent of finding an *equitable* solution. Effort is usually not expended examining the quality of the solution but rather on how well individuals will accept the solution.

Forcing

The forcing style of managing conflict is characterized by a supervisor seeking to meet his or her own goals at all costs, without concern for others' needs or whether they will accept the solution.[41] The supervisor sees losing as reducing status, weakness, and self-image; winning gives the supervisor a sense of achievement and power. Forcing suppresses conflict; issues that need thorough discussion generally are not raised. Since conflict is personalized by forcing, the issues are rarely dealt with objectively. This creates winners and losers. After repeated losses, employees may give up, having found that the environment is not conducive to collaborative and creative problem solving. The forcing style of conflict resolution often results in a win-lose solution.

Confronting

The confrontational approach to managing conflict is based on the perspective that conflict is an inherent part of organizational life. Therefore, ongoing conflict resolution processes must be developed, implemented, and periodically evaluated.

The supervisor or manager

1. Sees conflict as a natural part of the work environment that must be dealt with.
2. Feels that the attitudes and opinions of everyone need to be aired while confronting the conflict.
3. Recognizes that when a conflict is resolved to everyone's satisfaction, there will be more commitment to the solution reached.
4. Sees everyone in the organization as having an equal and important role in resolving conflict.[42]

Problems in the workplace are efficiently and effectively dealt with, both positive and negative information being shared by everyone involved. In solving the problem, employees recognize that their cooperation is essential if the goals in the workplace are to be met. Management teamwork is established by the mutual commitment of achieving agreed-upon goals and being able to work in an environment where collaboration is rewarded. This approach creates a win-win situation for everyone.

Although the confronting approach may seem time-consuming in the short run, it is time-conserving in the long run. It allows people to disagree but to work on their disagreements in light of the facts and ultimately to understand one another's point of view and the reasons for those views.

Although the confrontation style of achieving win-win solutions generally has been found most effective in managing conflict, there are situations in which another approach should be consciously and more effectively utilized. If anger prevents an employee from listening, then temporarily withdrawing that employee from the situation may be best. If an employee is angry, very verbal, and unwilling to listen to what anyone has to say, it may be best for the supervisor to listen (keeping in mind the employee's emotional state), withdraw, and maintain neutrality on the issue for the time being. This will give the employee an opportunity to calm down, to release frustration and some of the anger, and allow the supervisor an opportunity to provide an environment more conductive to win-win conflict resolution. Where the cause of a conflict appears to be lack of recognition or support, smoothing can be the most appropriate method. The employee who feels alone will get some comfort while the conflict is being resolved. A compromising approach might be the most viable method if the basic objective is immediate reduction of defensiveness. The supervisor, however, should not fall into the trap of finding an equitable solution rather than the best solution.

Effective conflict resolution, therefore, involves being able to reach a solution by identifying and defining the problem, discussing the problem, and arriving at a mutually acceptable solution. To achieve a win-win solution, the supervisor must

1. Have good communication skills, to help employees clarify the meaning of words and avoid misunderstandings. Most conflicts arise because of misunderstanding and individuals' jumping to the wrong conclusions. The supervisor must also realize that an employee's behavior and attitudes are influenced by the employee's emotional state, past experiences, and expectations brought to the conflict situation.
2. Be open and not defensive, and let employees know that their opinions are respected, using an approach that is not threatening.
3. Not perpetuate a gloom-and-doom attitude. Constant pessimism will lower employee morale and may make it more difficult to reach a win-win solution.
4. Acknowledge employees' achievements; proper compliments will help bring the employees together. Putting down employees accomplishments may create tension and escalate conflict.

Other forms of conflict resolution include mediation and arbitration. These are discussed in chapter 7.

CHAPTER 4 REFERENCES

1. Locke, E. A. "What Is Job Satisfaction?" *Organizational Behavior and Human Performance*, 4, 1969, 309–336.
2. Centers, R., and Bugental, D. "Intrinsic and Extrinsic Job Motivators Among Different Segments of the Working Population," *Journal of Applied Psychology*, 50, 1966, 193.
3. Morse, N., and Weiss, R. *"The Functions and Meaning of Work and the Job, American Sociology Review* 20, 1955, 191.
4. Weiss, B. "How to Manage the 'Creative' Person," *Management Review*, December 1974, 63, 37–40.
5. Weiss, B. Op. cit.

6. Smith, M.C. "Implications of 'Professionalization' for Pharmacy Education," American Journal Pharmacology Education, 34, February 1970, 16–32.
7. Disney, F. "Employee Turnover Is Costly," *Personnel Journal*, 33, 1954, 97.
8. Lvancevich, John M. "The Shortened Workweek: A Field Experiment," *Journal of Applied Psychology*, February 1977, 34–37.
9. Lublin, Joann. "The Four Day Week," *Wall Street Journal*, February 16, 1977.
10. Schneder, Harold. "Personnel Managers Look to the 80's," *Personnel Administrator*, November 1979, 47–53.
11. Buisman, Ben A. "4-Day, 40 Hour Work Week: Its Effects upon Labor Management," *Personnel Journal*, 54:11, November 1975, 566–567.
12. Holley, William, Jr., et al., "Employee Reactions to a Flex-time Program: A Longitudinal Study," *Human Resource Management*, Winter 1976.
13. Walton, Richard E. "Work Innovations in the United States," *Harvard Business Review*, 88–89, July-August 1979.
14. Morgan, Frank. "Your (Flex) Time May Come," *Personnel Journal*, February 1977, 82–85.
15. Olmstead, Barney. "Job Sharing—A New Way to Work," *Personnel Journal*, 56:2, February, 1977, 78–81.
16. Maslow, A.H. "A Theory of Human Motivation," *Psychological Review* 50, 1943, 370–396.
17. Maslow, A.H. *Motivation and Personality* (New York: Harper and Brothers, 1954).
18. McClelland, D.C., et al., *The Achievement Motive* (New York: Appleton-Century-Crofts, Inc., 1953).
19. Alderfer, C.P. *Existence, Relatedness and Growth Human Needs in Organizational Settings* (New York: The Free Press, 1972).
20. Herzberg, F.; Mausner, B.; and Synderman, B.; *The Motivation to Work*, 2nd ed. (New York: John Wiley and Sons, 1959).
21. House, R.J., and Wigdor, L.A. "Herzberg's Dual Factor Theory of the Evidence and a Criticism," *Personnel Psychology*, 20: 4, Winter 1967, 369–389.
22. Vroom, Victor H. *Work and Motivation* (New York: John Wiley and Sons, 1964).
23. Thorndike, E.L. *Animal Intelligence* (New York: MacMillian Publishing Co., 1911).

24. Rogers, Carl R., and Skinner, B.F. "Some Issues Concerning the Control of Human Behavior: A Symposium," *Science*, 124, November 1956, 1057–1066.

25. Locke, E.A. "Toward a Theory of Task Motivation and Incentives," *Organizational Behavior and Human Performance*, 3:2, May 1968, 157–189.

26. Latham, Gary, and Yukl, Gary. "A Review of the Research of the Application of Goal Setting in Organizations," *Academy of Management Journal*, 18:4, December 1975, 824–845.

27. Levinson, Harry. "Management by Whose Objectives?" *Harvard Business Review*, 48, 4, July-August 1970, 125–134.

28. Walton, R.E., and Dutton, J.M. "The Management of Interdepartmental Conflict: A Model and Review," *Administrative Science Quarterly*, 14, 1969, 73–84.

29. Walton, R.E.; Dutton, J.M.; and Cafferty, T.P. "Organizational Context and Interdepartmental Conflict," *Administrative Science Quarterly*, 14, 1969, 522–543.

30. Vroom, Victor H. "Industrial Social Psychology," In G. Lindsey, and E. Aronson, *Handbook of Social Psychology*, Vol. 5 (Reading, MA: Addison-Wesley, 1970), 239–240.

31. Maier, N.R. *Problem Solving Discussion and Conferences: Leadership Methods and Skills* (New York: McGraw-Hill, 1963).

32. Guetzkow, H., and Gyr, J. "An Analysis of Conflict in Decision-Making Groups," *Human Relations*, 7, 1954, 267–381.

33. Burke, R.J. "Methods of Resolving Superior-Subordinate Conflict: The Constructive Use of Subordinate Differences and Disagreements," *Organizational Behavior and Human Performance*, 5, 1970, 393–411.

34. Filley, A.C. *Interpersonal Conflict Resolution* (Glenview, IL: Scott Freman Co., 1975), 21–30.

35. Ibid., 23–24.

36. Burke, R.J. "Methods of Resolving Interpersonal Conflict," *Personnel Administrator*, 32, 1960, 48.

37. Filley, A.C. Op. cit.

38. Burke, R.J. Op. cit.

39. Blake, R., and Norton, J. *The Managerial Grid* (Houston, TX: Golf Publishing Co., 1975), 94.

40. Filley, A.C. Op. cit., 52.

41. Ibid., 51.

42. Ibid., 52.

Work and Health 5

The health of the management team (those in supervisory roles) and the employees will affect work productivity in any healthcare organizational setting. In private practice, the health of the practitioner is an important factor in maintaining a viable practice. This becomes even more important in solo practice.

Few, if any, individuals can perform effectively and efficiently when in poor health, frustrated, or burned out. Employers and supervisors should therefore assist all employees in dealing with these issues in the workplace should they occur, as well as guarding against them. This chapter will deal with work-related issues that can affect health (such as frustration, job burnout and stress) and their management.

Work can produce stress. Research indicates that psychological job stressors produce altered measurements of various bodily chemicals and organic functions, as well as altered levels of anxiety.[1,2,3]

The more hours worked above 40 per week, the higher an individual's risk for heart disease. Work overload produces psychological and physiological signs such as increased anxiety, tension, and an altered heart rate—all of which are risk factors in heart disease. Individuals working beyond 40 hours a week also have an increased risk of various types of accidents.

Friedman and Rosenman[4] identified a relationship between personality characteristics and the likelihood of having a heart attack. They identified two major behavior types: type A and type B. A type A individual is characterized as aggressive, hypercritical, thriving on tight deadlines, engaging in an incessant struggle to achieve more and more in less and less time, establishing very difficult goals, easily becoming impatient when goals and deadlines are not achieved, being status oriented, and never being satisfied with the symbols of achieved status. A type B individual, on the other hand, is more contemplative, takes time to weigh alternatives, is less status oriented, establishes longer time periods for achievement of goals, and is more patient when deadlines are not achieved.

The study concluded that in the absence of type A behavior, coronary heart disease almost never occurs before 70 years of age. Type As were not only three times more likely to develop heart disease than type Bs; type As who were low on other coronary risk factors were still more prone to heart disease than type Bs who smoked, were hypertensive, and whose family histories included heart attacks.

Individual susceptibility to job-related stress varies greatly. Increased stress at work and the presence of type A behavior can be detrimental not only to productivity but also to an individual's health. Employers therefore should not encourage type A behavior.

FRUSTRATION

Frustration develops in an individual who knows what he or she wants but is unable to achieve it because of perceived or real barriers. People become frustrated because the work environment prevents them from achieving their goals and getting the desired rewards. Frustration comes from a feeling of relative deprivation of goal achievement. Employee frustration is unhealthy in any work environment, yet we often hear people say they are frustrated with one thing or another. To effectively deal with frustration, it is essential to know what it is, what causes it, how to recognize it, and how to deal with it in the work environment.

Causes of Frustration

For most people, the healthy and mature reaction to a problem is problem-solving behavior. Problem solving involves variability and creativity when encountering an obstacle to one's goal. In problem solving, the individual may try to get around the obstacles. If, however, the obstacle is insurmountable, the individual may abandon the goal and settle for a substitute or a lesser goal. When goal abandonment or settling for an alternative goal is not possible, or there is high pressure for immediate goal achievement in spite of obstacles and any escape is blocked, an individual's failure may cause tension. The person may become frustrated rather than using effective problem-solving behavior. High or constant pressure, failure, and the inability to escape from a situation when a goal cannot be achieved given the circumstances will produce frustration. Frustration results from severe setbacks or continued hindrance or blocking of a desired endeavor. A frustrated person is under emotional tension; this, rather than the nature of the situation, determines behavior.[5] What, then, are some of the barriers or obstacles that block employees from reaching their goals? Some typical barriers in the workplace include the various forms of discrimination; insecurity; hostile, unsupportive supervisors; sexual harassment; personality conflicts; monotony in the job; unsafe working conditions; overall unpleasant working conditions; a lack of resources to get the job done; and assignments for which employees are unqualified or untrained (mismatched employees and jobs).

Discrimination

Discrimination may be based on race, gender, national origin, age, religion, disability, sexual orientation, political affiliation, or marital status. Federal law prohibits certain forms of discrimination in the workplace (these are discussed in chapter 7). Various state laws prohibit some forms of workplace discrimination not prohibited by federal law, so it is important to know what is prohibited in your own state. Any form of discrimination or favoritism among employees—such as reprimanding only certain employees for being late to work, or rewarding certain employees and ignoring others who should also be rewarded—may cause employee frustration. Discrimination in any form, even if not prohibited by law, should be avoided in the workplace to improve employee morale, productivity, and job satisfaction.

Insecurity

Employees who feel that their employment can be easily terminated regardless of their performance often become insecure. When employees are unsure of their position in a healthcare organization or unsure of their chances of promotion or upward mobility, these uncertainties may become a source of frustration.

Hostile, Unsupportive Supervisors

Where a supervisor or a manager is unsupportive or hostile, employees often become frustrated. A supportive supervisor does not necessarily agree with employees. Sometimes hostile behavior is a result of personality conflicts.

Sexual Harassment

Sexual harassment in the workplace is prohibited by law. Sexual harassment can include pictures, jokes, gestures, and any form of communication with a sexual connotation that is not welcomed by the individual to whom it is directed and makes that individual uncomfortable. Sexual harassment is discussed in chapter 7.

Personality Conflicts

When personality conflicts among employees remain unresolved, it can cause frustration. Conflict resolution to deal with personality problems is discussed in chapter 4.

Monotony in the Job

Doing the same thing day in, day out, with no variety, may not be a major problem in most healthcare organizations because most employees do have some level of interaction with patients, and this helps to introduce some variety to break the monotony.

Unsafe Working Conditions

Unsafe working conditions not only threaten employees' safety but may also cause employee frustration.

Unpleasant Working Conditions

No one likes to work in an uncomfortable environment. A working environment can be unpleasant if it is crowded, dirty, run down, or noisy. Lack of opportunity for advancement or self-fulfillment can be a form of unpleasant working conditions, and lead to lack of interest in a job.

Lack of Resources

Where the employer does not provide employees with the resources needed to complete a job, this will lead to frustration, especially if the employer still expects the job to be accomplished on time. Frustration may also occur where there are inadequate or unreliable resources for the employee to perform the job.

Mismatching an Employee and a Job

An employee may become frustrated if unable to effectively do the job. This occurs when an employee is neither qualified nor trained for an assignment. It is not unusual for employees to be promoted to positions for which they are inadequately prepared. They feel trapped in their new position because of their incompetency and inability to perform at the expected level.

Signs of Employee Frustration

What should an employer, supervisor, or manager look for to identify frustrated employees? An individual experiencing frustration feels tense and uncomfortable, a condition that may be referred to as anxiety. Anxiety and other signs of frustration are discussed below.

Anxiety may account for employee behavior that is often misunderstood and misinterpreted, such as resistance to change. Resistance to changes in work methods, work schedules, or new programs may occur because the individual feels threatened or frightened by the proposed changes. Anxiety sometimes leads to a supervisor's failure to delegate.

A frustrated individual usually engages in maladaptive behavior, such as aggression and hostility.[6] The absolute necessity of performing a task or the anticipation of punishment if the task is not completed before a deadline, creates a frustrating situation, and this may create a distinct change in behavior. What was previously healthy, unemotional activity now shows a degree of emotionality and unreasonableness. Constructive behavior is replaced by destructive behavior.[7]

Aggression is another symptom associated with frustration. Employee aggression typically involves verbal and physical attacks and hostile acts, and is often associated with anger. Some researchers have established a relationship between frustration and aggression.[8,9,10,11,12] When aggression against the individual causing the frustration is blocked, the angry person's energy may be directed at substitute objects[13] or individuals in the workplace or outside work, perhaps at home. When aggression is directed toward the frustrating agent or individual and the agent or individual strikes back, this results in further frustration rather than relief. Frustrated employees often show aggression and also tend to become defensive. To a frustrated individual, compliments paid by others may be seen as insults as the individual tends to become overly suspicious and paranoid. Aggression may result in problems with interpersonal relations, damage to equipment, harm to oneself, exposing other employees to dangerous situations, constant criticism, grievances, and absenteeism. The degree of aggressiveness exhibited by an individual as a result of frustration will vary from one person to another depending on personality traits, environmental factors, and the nature of the obstacle to goal achievement.

Regression, which is the breakdown of constructive behavior and the return to juvenile behavior, is another symptom of frustration.[14,15] When individuals are unable to act their age in problem situations, they are showing signs of regression. In the work environment these include loss of emotional control, pouting, forming blind loyalties to particular persons, or blindly following the leader. When intelligent people lose their perspective and fail to make objective distinctions, they have regressed.[16]

When all forms of activity seem closed, frustrated individuals often show signs of resignation or avoidance; literally, they give up. Resignation or avoidance may result in quitting the job or in a high rate of absenteeism. Those showing signs of resignation have lost all hope and feel that things will not get better in the work environment. They look forward to getting out of work. Such individuals often depress other employees with their feelings and statements of hopelessness, and their complaints of how terrible things are.

Another symptom of frustration is negativism. This can be defined as strong and irrational resistance to accepting the suggestions of others. An individual exhibiting negativism does not see anything good in the workplace or in other people in the healthcare organization. The individual who feels resigned will not see most activities as positive, instead showing strong and irrational resistance to accepting other people's suggestions. This individual objects to suggestions that originate from anyone else. The employee who shows signs of resignation becomes unreasonable, and seems always to make negative remarks about things going on in the workplace or about the management or administration. Even when things are improving, such individuals do not see the improvement.

A frustrated individual may also show signs of projection. The individual blames others for everything that goes wrong. Even when the individual should take the responsibility for what has gone wrong, he or she always finds someone else to blame. Individuals showing signs of projection refuse to take responsibility for even their own acts, because as far as they are concerned, it is always someone else's fault.

Signs of frustration are by no means limited to those discussed above. However, these are the most common signs. Whether an individual who is prevented from achieving a goal will develop symptoms of frustration depends on the individual's personality traits, personal experiences, and other factors, discussed below.

Some individuals are better able to tolerate barriers to strong goal achievement with minimal feelings of frustration because they have a higher degree of frustration tolerance. The development of frustration tolerance in individuals is not well understood; however, it seems to be influenced by early environmental experiences.[17]

What frustrates one individual may not frustrate another. Other determining factors in terms of developing symptoms of frustration are

- The individual's interpretation of the situation and the chances of eliminating the barrier, getting around the barrier so that the original goal can be achieved, or achieving an alternative but equally desirable goal.
- The individual's personal preparation for the frustrating situation—the more prepared an individual is for a potentially frustrating situation, the better able he or she will be to handle it.
- The individual's previous history of frustration.
- The time pressure under which employees are performing. The more time they have to deal with a problem, the more effectively they will handle it.
- The barriers blocking the individual from achieving a desired goal. Interference caused by other people within or outside the work environment seems more likely to produce frustration than does interference caused by a physical object.
- The individual's culture.
- Previous experience in handling the frustrating situation.
- The ability to cope with problem situations.

Dealing With Employee Frustration

In handling frustration, one should not lose sight of the fact that individual variations exist. Not everybody will react exactly the same way when frustrated. Frustrated individuals can exhibit differently any of the symptoms. Some employees may show one symptom or a combination of symptoms when frustrated. As indicated earlier, differences in individual responses to frustration can be attributed to cultural differences, previous experiences, ability to cope with problem situations, and personality differences. Although individual differences exist, an understanding of basic behavioral changes will enable supervisors, employers, and employees to deal more effectively with frustrations in the workplace.

The first step in dealing with frustration is barrier identification. In preventing or dealing with frustration it is very important to identify the frustrating obstacle or barrier to goal achievement. Open communication and good communication skills are the key to barrier identification. Discussing the problem with the employee will help identify the obstacle to the employee's goal achievement in the workplace. The employee must be comfortable enough with the supervisor to identify barriers without fear of retaliation, especially if the barrier is another individual in the workplace or even the supervisor.

The second step is analysis of the identified barrier. The supervisor or manager must identify its nature and find potential solutions to the problem. This step depends on the first step—one cannot find a solution to a barrier unless one knows the nature of the barrier and to what extent the barrier is preventing goal achievement.

The final step is removing the obstacle, getting around the obstacle, or creating an alternative but equally desirable and achievable goal. By identifying, analyzing, and removing barriers to goal achievement, or by enabling employees to achieve alternative goals, the supervisor or manager creates a work environment that enables individuals to work toward professional and organizational goals,[18] and toward personal growth.

JOB BURNOUT

The term "burnout" means different things to different people—it is easier to describe than to define. In general, it refers to a loss of physical and mental energy as a result of constant work pressure, which drains the individual. The term is applied most frequently in the work arena. Freudenberger[19] was one of the pioneers in the area of job burnout. Research has indicated that burnout occurs among various personnel, including those in healthcare.[20,21,22,23,24] Burnout undermines the morale and well-being of the healthcare employee, which may have a negative impact on the quality of care given to patients.

Job Burnout Defined

Job burnout is sometimes equated with job stress. Although they may be related, they are not synonymous. Burnout may be a consequence of job stress. An individual may experience job stress and not burn out; however, an individual usually will not burn out without experiencing job stress.

There are various definitions of burnout. Veninga and Spradley[25] defined burnout as a debilitating psychological condition brought about by unrelieved work stress causing

1. Depleted energy reserves.
2. Lowered resistance to illness.
3. Increased dissatisfaction and pessimism.
4. Increased absenteeism and inefficiency at work.

In this definition, burnout is seen as a direct consequence of continuous job stress, thus implying a direct cause-and-effect relationship.

Maslach[26] in her definition characterized burnout as a term common to people in human services. She defined burnout as the loss of concern for the people with whom one is working; it is characterized by exhaustion and by loss of positive feelings, respect, or sympathy for clients or patients.[27] The individual becomes detached from clients or patients, in contrast to a previously positive attitude toward the work environment.

Pines and Aronson defined burnout as "the result of constant or repeated emotional pressure associated with intense involvement with people over long periods of time."[28] They also viewed burnout as a state of mind affecting people who give more to clients, colleagues, and supervisors than they receive from those people. These researchers suggested that burnout involves mental, physical, and emotional fatigue; loss of enthusiasm and interest; and feelings of helplessness and hopelessness. Burnout, therefore, affects those professionals who were once the most idealistic, energetic and enthusiastic individuals.

Edelwich and Brodsky restricted their use of the term to the helping professions, and maintained that burnout occurs more in the human services professions, with higher social costs, even though it can occur in any profession. They defined burnout as "a progressive loss of idealism, energy and purpose experienced by people in the helping professions as a result of the conditions of their work."[29] It is, therefore, the stressful nature of the human services work environment that tends to increase health professionals' vulnerability to burnout, compared to other professionals.

Cherniss defined burnout as a "process in which a previously committed professional disengages from his or her work in response to stress and strain experienced on the job."[30] In this definition job stress is again seen as a prerequisite to burnout in a previously committed individual. It also appears that the strong altruistic humanitarian commitment of healthcare employees makes them more vulnerable to burnout. This same line of thought can be seen in Muldary's definition of burnout as the process by "which a once-committed health professional becomes ineffective in managing the stress of frequent emotional contact with others in the helping context, experiences exhaustion and as a result, disengages from patients, colleagues and the organization." [31]

These definitions point out some generally accepted aspects of burnout:

1. Burnout is related to work stress.
2. It is related to continuous pressures in the work environment.
3. It occurs more often in the helping professions.
4. It negatively affects the client or patient and other individuals with whom or for whom the burned-out person works.
5. It has serious consequences, such as exhaustion, disengagement, decreased productivity, and lowered resistance to illness.

In this textbook, burnout is defined as a consequence of unmanaged or poorly managed sustained stress, brought about by interaction with the work environment and the individual's strong, unselfish commitment to helping others, which results in abnormal physical, emotional, mental, or behavioral signs or symptoms.

Job burnout occurs in both employees and employers who are idealistic, enthusiastic high achievers—individuals who want to accomplish tasks and be successful in their professional career. One of the major causes of job burnout is organizational pressure associated with work. Individuals do not burn out overnight. An employer or employee burns out as a result of continuous work overload. Individuals have varying burnout thresholds.

Signs and Symptoms

Burned out individuals wake up tired—exhausted even though they may have slept for 10 hours. This may happen because the exhaustion is mental and they feel run down. They may become angry about the way things are going at work, which sooner or later affects their personal life. They may become paranoid and may develop physiological symptoms such as fatigue, high blood pressure, sleeplessness, anxiety, and ulcers. Their bodies find a way to tell them to slow down. The burned-out individual also goes through behavioral changes, possibly becoming irritable and losing a sense of humor and enthusiasm.

Although burnout is a multidimensional syndrome, unyielding to simplistic analysis, the validity of the term becomes diluted when it is viewed in such a way that virtually everything is included as a cause, symptom, or consequence. To better understand burnout it is important that etiological explanations consider the fact that some people burn out but others do not, even when exposed to the same or worse conditions. The individualistic nature of burnout must be recognized as a function of the individual's relationship and coping ability. Individuals in the late stages of burnout show signs of job disappointment, disillusionment, and despair.

Burnout has a vast range of symptoms and seems to be a highly variable combination of behaviors, attitudes, and symptoms.[32] These include

- Job dissatisfaction.
- Loss of sense of humor.
- Tiredness or fatigue.
- Boredom.
- Sleeping problems.
- Cynicism.
- Loss of enthusiasm.
- Resignation.
- Headaches.
- Low morale.
- Psychosomatic illness.
- Lack of confidence.
- Tension.
- Difficulty concentrating.
- Obnoxiousness.
- Fault finding.
- Nausea.
- Defensiveness.
- Weight problems.
- Isolation and withdrawal.
- Increased accidents.
- Loss of empathy.
- Irritability.
- Stereotyping of patients.
- Anxiety.
- Absenteeism.
- Paranoia.
- Increased mistakes.
- Apathy.
- Clock watching.
- Feelings of guilt.
- Tardiness.
- Anger.
- Conflict with others (work and family).
- Suicidal thoughts.
- Feelings of being trapped.
- Resentment.
- Unnecessary risk taking.
- Frustration.
- Use of drugs and alcohol to cope.
- Disillusionment.

Although burnout can occur in any occupation, it seems more prevalent among people whose jobs involve helping others and require frequent emotional contact with people. This may be a result of the intense, constant involvement with distressed, sick, and ill people.

Dealing With Job Burnout

1. The employer or supervisor should give the employee some time off for a vacation. Being too busy to take a vacation may be a warning sign of burnout. Two short vacations are usually better than one long one.
2. Exercise will help to relieve work-related stress and therefore reduce the chances of job burnout.
3. Cut down time at work to no more than 45 hours a week. If necessary, the manager should hire another person to help with the workload, rather than constantly overloading an employee.
4. Set realistic job and time schedules; do not try to be a superman or superwoman, or make others superpeople.
5. Supervisors should select the right jobs for themselves and their employees.
6. Recognition of the symptoms is an important step in dealing with job burnout.
7. If all else fails, the affected individual should be moved to a different work area, if possible.

STRESS MANAGEMENT
by Anthony Wutoh, Ph.D.

Introduction

In the daily workplace of a healthcare professional, stress is inevitable, unavoidable, and often a constant source of frustration. The key to a productive and healthy workplace is not simply the avoidance of stress but also the effective management of stressful situations as they occur. Stress is a major problem in the United States; the economic impact of lost productivity as a result of stress is virtually incalculable. In 1988, it was estimated that stress disorders cost U.S. industries as much as $150 billion a year in decreased productivity.[33] Research has identified a correlation between stress and the incidence of hypertension, myocardial infarction, headaches, mental disorders, and a host of other health-related concerns.[34,35,36,37] The costs of these and other ailments related to stress has also been on the rise. As early as the mid-1960s, cardiovascular disease accounted for 12 percent of all missed workdays, at a cost of $4 billion in lost productivity.[38] In the 1970s, the medical cost of recurrent headaches was $1.2 billion, and they cost another $6.2 billion in lost productivity.[39]

It has been estimated that as much as 50 percent of worker absenteeism may be stress related. [40] In short, a healthy lifestyle means more than just the absence of disease; an environment in which stress is controlled and dealt with in a productive manner is as essential to good health as the availability of medical care.

Definitions of Stress

Beehr and Newman defined job stress as a condition arising from the interaction of people and their jobs and characterized by changes within people that force them to deviate from their normal functioning. [41] This definition is best conceptualized by viewing the body and mind of an individual in a state of equilibrium. As a result of a stressor, that equilibrium is disrupted, and the individual functions differently in addressing various situations while in this state of disequilibrium. Others define stress as a physical and psychological consequence of any demand on a person or as an emotional by-product of any threat to a person. Reactions to stress are not localized; they may occur in various parts of the body. Stress may present itself as muscle tension, headache, nausea, hypertension, or sweating. Psychological manifestations of stress are also prevalent; they include anxiety, fear, depression, irritability, and worry. [42]

Many scientists believe that our physical reactions to stress are merely a by-product of the prehistoric *fight or flight* response that enabled early humans to address stressful, life-threatening situations. When a stressor is encountered, muscles often become tensed as glucose is released; this may result in neck and lower back pain, headaches, and grinding of teeth. Breathing becomes more rapid and shallow to allow for more rapid metabolization of glucose. Heart rate and blood pressure increase to improve the delivery of glucose around the body. Further, digestion is slowed to a standstill, which is why extreme stress is often associated with nausea and vomiting or upset stomachs. Finally, the body perspires more in an attempt to cool itself from the increased expenditure of energy associated with stress. [43]

The role of stress in the development of illness has been observed for many years, but it is only during the past 50 years that science has gained a significant understanding of how it affects people. The systematic investigation of stress began in the early 1920s with the findings of William B. Cannon and other physiologists, who studied the body's response to emotional stimuli. [44] This work initiated the study of hormonal and chemical mediators and their role in the body's adaptation to internal and external environmental changes. In the 1930s, Alexander and Dunbar observed a relationship between distinctive personality patterns and their predisposition to various "organic disorders." [45] The psychosomatic theory of disease was a result of these early observations. Simply stated, the theory holds that personality patterns and emotional response to various stimuli predispose people to particular patterns of illness.

In 1936, Hans Selye defined stress as the "nonspecific response of the body to any demand"; he further defined a stressor as any agent that produces stress at any time. [46] Dodge and Martin, in 1970, defined stress as a product of specific socially structured situations inherent in the organization of modern technological societies. [47] More recent investigation has added to our knowledge and led to the identification of "risk factors" for the development of stress. Risk factors are characteristics that influence a person's susceptibility to a particular illness. While an individual's association with one or more risk factors does not definitely ensure development of a particular illness, it does suggest that there is greater risk than for an individual who does not have that factor.

Stress Management

The goal of stress-management programs is to reduce the negative effects of stress-related work and personal problems on individuals at risk for developing stress. Therefore, it is essential in a program of stress management to first identify individuals who may need help at one point or another. The very existence of a stress-management program is instrumental in that it recognizes the importance of stress as a potential concern.

Various strategies and programs have been developed to address stress. These include group therapy, organizational restructuring, exercise and nutritional programs, career counseling, and a host of others. Key to any strategy is the identification of employees at risk for stress-related complications and the accessibility of one or more strategies to address stress, both in the workplace and in personal life. When not addressed, stress ultimately results in a decrease in organizational effectiveness. This may be manifested as reduction in quality, productivity, efficiency, profit, growth, or stability. It may also result in an increase in employee dissatisfaction, turnover, absenteeism, or drug and alcohol abuse.

Stress has a direct effect on the quality of working life. Walton, in 1973, identified eight aspects of work that, viewed together, determine the quality of working life. They are

1. Adequate and fair compensation.
2. Safe and healthy working conditions.
3. The immediate opportunity to use and develop human capacities.
4. Opportunity for continued growth and security.
5. Social integration in the work organization.
6. Constitutionalism in work organizations.
7. A balanced work role.
8. Social responsibility of the work organization.[48]

It is easy to see how the absence of one or more of these factors may lead to an increase in worker dissatisfaction, frustration, and stress. These determinants of the quality of work life can aid in the development of a listing of potential sources of stress.

Sources of Stress

During the course of a day there are many potential sources of stress; the list below enumerates only a few:

- Pleasant events.
- Unpleasant events.
- Changes of any kind.
- Attitudes and beliefs.
- Anticipation.
- Conflicts of any kind.
- Inability to resolve past events, feelings of guilt or self-pity.
- Intense noise.
- Inability to hear without straining.
- Extreme hot or cold temperatures.
- Illness of any kind, affecting the individual or someone close.
- Commuting on an unreliable system.
- Driving in heavy traffic.

There are also many potential sources of job-related stress. A general listing of job-related sources of stress includes

- Ambiguous or conflicting roles.
- Responsibility but little control.
- Minimal support from supervisors or subordinates.
- Lack of recognition or praise.
- Lack of opportunity for self-expression or creativity.
- Too much work; too little time.

- Poor performance by subordinates, peers, or managers.
- Tough quality standards; performance evaluations.
- Strain from the work schedule.
- Fear of failure, and consequent reduction in self-esteem.
- The office environment (office politics and cliques, for example).
- Communication problems.
- Job dissatisfaction.[49]

This general list demonstrates that everyone is potentially at risk for development of stress-related problems. A.P. Brief and colleagues grouped job-related stresses into three major categories: organizational characteristics and processes; job demands and role characteristics; and individual characteristics and expectations.[50] Organizational characteristics and processes include issues related to organizational policies such as pay inequities; organizational structure, including issues such as size and centralization; and organizational processes, which include communication issues and training programs. Job demands include issues such as working conditions, interpersonal relationships, and role issues. Individual characteristics include expectations and goals, job insecurity, flexibility, and other personal issues.

Increased organizational size leads to more sophisticated social structuring, which can result in greater stress. A centralized organizational structure can also contribute to feelings of a lack of participation in decision making, which can result in alienation and stress. There may be various other sources of job stress; this is merely an overview of the topic. Several evaluations have been developed to help identify both sources of stress and the effect of stress on an individual. The next two pages have a sample stress checklist to aid in recognition of symptoms of stress.

Personal Mechanisms for Coping With Job Stress

Several individual characteristics are influential in predicting responses to stress. The most profound of these are personality traits—for example, whether a person is introverted or extroverted can have great influence on the person's response to a stressor.[51] Introverted people are generally less likely to be expressive of their emotions and are more sensitive to their environments.[52] Many researchers feel that introverts are more likely to respond negatively to stress. Another factor that has been researched in terms of response to stress is locus of control. Internally oriented people believe that rewards and life consequences are within their control.[53] On

A Stress Checklist

_____ I become upset over little worries.

_____ I change my mind; I'm indecisive.

_____ I become bored; nothing excites me.

_____ I can't concentrate.

_____ I become cranky and irritable.

_____ I misjudge people.

_____ I feel dissatisfied.

_____ I can't sleep.

_____ I put things off.

_____ I have no energy.

_____ I can't eat.

_____ I eat too much.

_____ I lose weight.

_____ I gain weight.

_____ I smoke more.

_____ I drink more alcohol.

_____ I don't socialize.

_____ I feel my heart racing.

_____ I perspire more.

_____ My body aches.

_____ I grind my teeth.

_____ I feel tired in the afternoon.

_____ I am more distrustful.

_____ My confidence has eroded.

_____ I can't relax and do nothing.

_____ I work too much.

_____ I have no interest in sex.

_____ I find it hard to show emotion.

_____ I feel numb in emotional situations.

_____ I am intolerant of specific people, places, or things.

_____ I overreact.

_____ I feel like a time bomb about to explode.[54]

These are common responses to stress; none are good or bad, right or wrong.

_____ Do you see any patterns in your body's stress behavior?

Another example of a self-evaluation is the "Simple Stress and Tension Test" presented below.

A Simple Stress and Tension Test[55]

	Often	A few times a week	Rarely
I feel tense, anxious, or have nervous indigestion.			
People at work or home arouse my anger.			
I eat, drink, or smoke in response to tension.			
I have tension or migraine head-aches, pain in the neck or shoulders, or insomnia.			
I can't turn off my thoughts at night or on weekends long enough to feel relaxed or refreshed the next day.			
I find it difficult to concentrate on what I'm doing because of worrying about other things.			
I take tranquilizers or other drugs to relax.			
I have difficulty finding enough time to relax.			
Once I find the time, it's hard for me to relax.	(Yes)	(No)	
My workday is made up of too many deadlines.	(Yes)	(No)	

Responses to self-evaluations such as these help identify individuals who are under stress or who may be at risk for stress-related complications.

J.W. Farquhar, *The American Way of Life Need Not Be Hazardous to Your Health,* © 1987 Stanford Alumni Association. Reprinted by permission of Addison-Wesley Publishing Company, Inc.

the other hand, externally oriented people believe that life consequences are not within their control and that they are subject to the will of external forces. Because internally oriented people tend to be very much in control of life situations, they become very stressed when they feel that control over a given situation has been wrested from them, whereas externally oriented people believe in fate and luck, and are more anxious when forced to take control over the occurrence of stressful events. "Internals" generally experience less job stress and respond better functionally than "externals".[56]

Several other personality traits have been related to response to stress, including the ability of an individual to be flexible in situations, authoritarianism and dogmatism in terms of adherence to various moral beliefs, and ability to adapt to new situations. Personality traits help determine what strategies an individual adopts in response to stress. Strategies for coping with stress have been grouped into two categories: direct action and palliation. Direct action includes several approaches toward stress, such as preparing against danger, aggression, avoidance, and inaction. Palliation involves symptom-reduction methods, which may include both external agents such as alcohol and drug use or internal-control techniques such as muscle relaxation.[57]

Personal mechanisms for dealing with stress include both direct action and palliation techniques. The most commonly used relaxation technique is meditation.[58] This involves sustained concentration on an idea, object, or single word. This technique is thought to act through restriction of mental and physical activity. While meditation is often associated with mysticism or religious philosophies, there are various techniques that focus strictly on mental concentration and relaxation. Biofeedback is another mechanism for coping with stress. It involves the use of instruments to monitor physical processes involved with stress response, including blood pressure, heart rate, muscle tension, and breathing.[59] It is believed that this feedback is instrumental in enabling an individual to become more active in managing responses to stress. Meditation and biofeedback can be, and often are, used in conjunction to manage stress.

Another mechanism for coping with job stress is psychodynamic therapy. This form of therapy is designed to help people obtain deeper insight into the psychodynamic processes involved with stress, and their responses to stressors.[60] Freudian psychoanalysis and encounter groups are two forms of this type of therapy. Behavioral therapy includes techniques such as self-reinforcement and behavioral modification. Behavioral therapy differs from psychodynamic therapy in that less emphasis is placed on gaining insight into the root cause of stress problems, and greater emphasis is focused on altering future behavior patterns.[61] Self-reinforcement allows people to establish standards for their own behavior and the way that they will respond to stressful situations. As people successfully deal with stressful events, they may treat themselves with special rewards.[62]

The final personal technique to be discussed is planning. Planning involves taking a look at future events and identifying goals and potential stressors, and developing methods for achieving those goals while minimizing the negative stressors associated with the goals. This method involves a simple four-step process:

1. Define the problem.
2. Critically assess your personal resources to deal with the problem.
3. Select an appropriate coping mechanism.
4. Evaluate the effect of applying the coping mechanism.[63]

This methodology requires constant self-evaluation of capabilities and abilities to cope with various situations. It also involves regular reassessment to evaluate the effectiveness of applying a particular coping technique. One potential drawback of this approach is the possible inappropriateness of the coping mechanism selected. A coping mechanism such as escapism (the complete avoidance of dealing with problems) would work to reduce stress immediately, but it would serve only to postpone another stressful event.

Organizational Stress-Management Programs

Stress management has become an integral part of worksite health promotional strategies. In 1988, approximately 27 percent of worksites had some type of stress-management activity. The prevalence of stress-management programs increased with the number of employees. While 60 percent of companies with more than 250 employees had a stress-management program, only 15 percent of those with fewer than 100 employees had such a program.[64] In an effective stress-management program, the employee is the client.

The goals of a stress-management program are to increase people's skills at managing life stress and to provide help to people with special problems. Heirich (1988) determined that there are three crucial elements in ensuring the success of a stress-management program. First, follow-up is absolutely essential. In programs where staff was provided for follow-up, there was 50 percent to 90 percent employee participation, whereas in programs without one-to-one outreach, there was lower participation—from 1 percent to 10 percent. Second, most employees are not interested in health education classes to change behavior; there is greater interest in guided self-help programs. Therefore, wellness programs cannot rely on health education classes as their primary means of changing behavior. Third, social support systems are essential to the success of stress management.[65] Behavioral change and adjustment require support from a network of family, friends, or coworkers.

Heirich further concluded that there are four lessons to be learned from the establishment of a stress-management program: first, any method for health improvement must be actively introduced to employees; second, all approaches should be introduced in simple, incremental steps; third, a program must deal realistically with immediate problems and offer short-term benefits; fourth, in order for health improvement to become habitual, there must be regular follow-up and reminders of a commitment to better health.

Organizational Strategies for Stress Management

Five major types of stress-management programs have been used to help employees manage stress and to minimize its negative consequences: These stress management programs are: educational/awareness building, assessment-focused, skill-building (focusing on relaxation, coping, and interpersonal skills), therapeutic/counseling, and organizational/environmental change.[66] The type of program adopted by an employer is determined by several major aspects of the organization:

1. Organizational structure.
2. Relationships in the organization.
3. Roles in the organization.
4. Change.
5. Physical environment.
6. Career development.
7. Intrinsic job qualities.

While establishing the program the following goals should be established: (1) senior management's increased awareness of stress in their organization and its relationship to insurance losses; (2) feedback from the research team to senior managers on their assessment of the sources and levels of stress; (3) identification of high-risk groups or units, along with personal consultations to correct underlying problems; (4) establishment of an employee assistance program to provide ongoing psychological services to employees and their families for work- and non–work-related problems; and (5) various health programs, typically including stress-management training and education, inducements to exercise, healthful lifestyle advice, and avoidance of stress-related back injuries.

Though organizational stress-management programs may take many forms and involve various types of stress-reduction and stress-avoidance techniques, Pelletier (1988) made the following recommendations regarding individualized programs: (1) identification of symptomatic and high-risk individuals; (2) thorough evaluation of those individuals by qualified health professionals; (3) appropriate referral and treatment of motivated individuals; (4) treatment provided by professionals skilled with brief intervention protocols; (5) appropriate follow-up to ensure maintenance of treatment; (6) health and cost-effectiveness evaluation on a regular and ongoing basis. Further, packaged programs should take place once a week for four to eight weeks; sessions should take 45 minutes; and the ideal group size is between 12 and 15.[67]

While there are costs involved in the establishment of an organizational stress-management program, the potential savings from improvments in worker efficiency, morale, and attendance will be cost-effective. In 1988, the cost of worker absenteeism, including lost productivity, was $150 billion.[68] It is easy to see how improved mental health and stress reduction at work could result in improved occupational production.

Personal Strategies for Stress Management

There are several steps that an individual can take to reduce or prevent stress; everyday activities such as exercise, relaxation, and proper diet can make remarkable differences in physical and mental health. In terms of nutrition, a well-balanced diet including fruits, vegetables, and grains is essential to proper health. Some advocates of nutritional programs for stress reduction have suggested that special diets may relieve symptoms of stress; others have suggested that stress places extra demands on the body, thereby requiring the ingestion of "anti-stress factors," including vitamins and minerals. While research has not adequately addressed these theories, it is clear that "junk food" is not good for nutrition and is likely to inhibit the body's ability to cope with stress.[69]

The benefits of exercise have been demonstrated—it reduces blood pressure, reduces the risk of stroke, improves circulation, and generally improves the health of the body. Exercise as a form of release is key to an overall stress-reduction strategy.[70] Recreational activities that promote group involvement, along with team games, are also effective in building teamwork and providing opportunities to relieve stress. The benefits of meditation and relaxation techniques have been known for a very long time. In some form or another, relaxation techniques have been practiced by every known culture. From ritual prayer and incantations to Transcendental Meditation, meditation can play a major role in stress reduction.[71]

Proponents of biofeedback training feel that, since the mind and body are clearly interrelated, self-regulation of physiological functions leads to increased self-awareness, which then helps people deal with their problems. With sufficient training, people can be trained to regulate their heart rate, blood pressure, and other physiological functions to the point at which stress is greatly reduced or avoided entirely.[72,73]

Career counseling is a valuable alternative for individuals who are in jobs for which they are ill suited or in which they see no future. Dissatisfaction with employment can be a very great source of stress; however, there are situations in which organizational programs and other personal strategies will have little effect. It is important for individuals to know that there are alternatives to their current employment—alternatives that will take full advantage of their skills and talents while providing meaningful benefit to society. There are also several group approaches to stress management; these include group therapy and psychoanalysis but may also be informally structured as rap sessions or social clubs for the mutual benefit of the members.

There are several key components to stress management as a lifestyle, including

1. Finding new interests.
2. Actively working to avoid unnecessary stress.
3. Managing time more successfully.
4. Not worrying about things that cannot be controlled.
5. Getting enough restful sleep.[74]

There are various other things that can be incorporated into the daily schedule to manage stress. These include walking more often, seeking advice about sexual or emotional problems, developing a hobby, concentrating on the current task, finishing one thing before starting another, avoiding impossible deadlines or other promises, learning to express feelings openly, accepting personal responsibility for one's life and health, and, finally, greeting, smiling at, and responding to people in the manner in which one would like to be treated.

Humans are social beings. It is important to develop and maintain a support network of family, friends, coworkers, neighbors, and other people who will interact and help to maintain a healthy emotional environment. It is also essential to remember the role of humor and laughter in our lives. Laughter is great medicine. The effect of a good laugh to relieve tension can be felt immediately. It is often good not to take life too seriously.

CHAPTER 5 REFERENCES

1. Levi, Lennart. *Stress, and Distress in response to Psychosocial Stimuli; Laboratory and real-life studies on Sympatho-adreno-medullary and related reactions.* Edited by Lennart Levi, Pergamon Press, N.Y. 1972.

2. Hinkle, L.E., Jr., "The Concept of 'Stress' in the Biological and Social Sciences," *International Journal of Psychiatry in Medicine*, 5:4, 1974, 335–337, 355–356.

3. Levi, Lennant. *Stress, Sources, Management and Prevention.* (New York: Leverright, 1967).

4. Friedman, M., and Rosenman, R.H. *Type A: Your Behavior and Your Heart* (New York: Knopf, 1974).

5. Maier, Norman R.F. *Frustration* (Ann Arbor, MI: University of Michigan Press, 1961).

6. Chruden, Herbert J., and Sherman, Arthur W. *Personnel Management* (Dallas, TX: Southwestern Publishing Company, 1980).

7. Ibid.

8. Dollard, J., et al. *Frustration and Aggression* (New Haven, CT: Yale University Press, 1961).

9. McNeio, E.C., "Psychology and Aggression," *Journal of Conflict Resolution*, 3, 1959, 195–293.

10. Scott, J.P. *Aggression.* (Chicago: University of Chicago Press, 1958).

11. Sears, P.S. "Doll Play Aggression in Young Children," *Psychological Monograph*, 65, 1951.

12. Freshback, S. "Dynamics and Morality of Violence and Aggression— Some Psychological Considerations," *American Psychologist*, 26, 1971, 281–292.

13. Watson, G.A. "Comparison of the Effects of Lax Versus Strict Home Training," *Journal of Social Psychology*, 5, 1934, 105.

14. Baker, R.; Demo, T.; and Lewin, K. *Frustration and Regression* (Iowa City, IA: University of Iowa Press, 1942).

15. Baruch, D.W. "Therapeutic Procedures as Part of the Educational Process," *Journal of Consultation Psychology*, 4, 1940, 165–172.

16. Maier, Norman R.F. *Psychology in Industrial Organizations*, 4th ed. (Boston: Houghton Mifflin Company, 1973).

17. Chruden, Herbert J., and Sherman, Arthur W. Op. cit.

18. Wilkens, Paul L., and Haynes, Joel B. "Understanding Frustration— Instigated Behavior," *Personnel Journal*, 53; 10, 770–774.

19. Freudenberger, H.J., "Staff Burnout," *Journal of Social Issues*, 30, 1974, 159–165.

20. Hall, R.C.W.; Gardner, E.R.; Perl, M.; Stickney, S.K.; and Pfefferbarum, B. "The Professional Burnout Syndrome," *Psychiatric Opinion*, 16, (4) 1979, 12–13, 16–17.

21. Pines, A., and Aronson, E. *Burnout: From Tedium to Personal Growth* (New York: Free Press, 1981).

22. Pines, A., and Maslach, C. "Characteristics of Staff Burnout in Mental Health Settings," *Hospital and Community Psychiatry*, 29, 1978, 233–237.

23. Veninga, R.L., and Spradley, J.P. *The Work Stress Connection: How to Cope with Job Burnout* (Boston: Little, Brown, 1981).

24. LaVandero, R. "Nurse Burnout: What Can We Learn?" *Journal of Nursing Administration*, 12 (11) 1981, 17–23.

25. Veninga, R.L., and Spradley, J.P. Op. cit., 6.

26. Maslach, C., and Jackson, S.E. "Lawyer Burnout," *Barrister*, 5 (2), 1977, 52–54.

27. Ibid.

28. Pines, A., and Aronson, E. Op. cit., 15.

29. Edelwich, J., and Brodsky, A. *Burnout: Stages of Disillusionment in the Helping Professions* (New York: Human Sciences Press, 1980), 14.

30. Cherniss, C. *Staff Burnout: Job Stress in the Human Service* (Beverly Hills, CA: Sage Publications, 1980), 18.

31. Muldary, T.W. *Burnout and Health Professionals: Manifestations and Management* (Norwalk, CT: Appleton-Century-Crofts, 1983), 12.

32. LaVandero, R. Op. cit.

33. Frecknall, P. "How Much Can Mind-Body Techniques Save by Reducing Absenteeism?" *Advances*, 6, 1989, 63–65.

34. Charlesworth, E.; Williams, B.; Baer, P. "Stress Management at the Work Site for Hypertension: Compliance, Cost-Benefit, Health Care, and Hypertension-Related Variables," *Psychosomatic Medicine*, 46, 1984, 387–97.

35. Blanchard, E.; Andrasik, F.; Appelbaum, K.A.; et al. "The Efficacy and Cost-Effectiveness of Minimal-Therapist-Contact, Non-Drug Treatments of Chronic Migraine and Tension Headache," *Headache*, 25, 1985, 214–19.

36. Ost, L. "Applied Relaxation: Description of a Coping Technique and Review of Controlled Studies," *Behavior Residence Therapy*, 25, 1987, 397–409.

37. Glass, D.C. *Behavior Patterns, Stress, and Coronary Disease* (Hillsdale, NJ: John Wiley, 1977).
38. Felton, J.S., and Cole, R. "The High Cost of Heart Disease," *Circulation*, 27, 1963, 957–62.
39. Jones, J., and Dosedel, J. "The Impact of Corporate Stress Management on Insurance Losses," *Legal Insight*, 1, 1986, 24–7.
40. Bureau of National Affairs. Personnel Policies Forum Survey, 132, 1984, 3–11.
41. Beehr, T.A., and Newman, J.E. "Job Stress, Employee Health, and Organizational Effectiveness: A Facet Analysis, Model, and Literature Review," *Personnel Psychology*, 31, 665–99.
42. Warshaw, L.J. *Managing Stress* (Reading, MA: Addison-Wesley, 1979).
43. U.S. Department of Health and Human Services. *Federal Ex-stress: When You Need Relief Overnight—A Stress Management Guide*, 1988.
44. Warshaw, L.J. Op. cit.
45. Ibid.
46. Selye, H. "A Syndrome Produced by Diverse Nocuous Agents," *Nature*, 138, 1936, 32.
47. Dodge, D., and Martin, W. *Social Stress and Chronic Illness* (Notre Dame, IN: University of Notre Dame Press, 1970).
48. Walton, R.E. "Quality of Working Life: What Is It?" *Sloan Management Review*, 1973, 11–21.
49. U.S. Department of Health and Human Services. *Federal Ex-stress.*
50. Brief, A.P.; Aldag, R.J.; Van Sell, M.; et al. "Anticipatory Socialization and Role Stress Among Registered Nurses," *Journal of Health and Social Behavior*, 20, 1979, 161–66.
51. Wilson, G.D., "Personality," in H.S. Eysenck and G.D. Wilson, eds., *A Textbook in Human Psychology* (Baltimore: University Park Press, 1976).
52. Kahn, R.L.; Wolfe, D.M.; Quinn, R.R.; et al. *Organizational Stress: Studies in Role Conflict and Ambiguity* (New York: Wiley, 1964).
53. Houston, B.K. "Control Over Stress, Locus of Control, and Response to Stress," *Journal of Personality and Social Psychology*, 21, 1972, 249–55.
54. U.S. Department of Health and Human Services. *Federal Ex-stress.*
55. Farquhar, J.W. (© 1987 Stanford Alumni Association) *The American Way of Life Need not Be Hazardous to Your Health* (Reading, MA: Addison-Wesley Publishing Co., Inc., 1987).

56. Anderson, C.R. "Locus of Control, Coping Behaviors, and Performance in a Stress Setting: A Longitudinal Study," *Journal of Applied Psychology*, 62, 1977, 4446–51.

57. Lazarus, R.S. *Psychological Stress and the Coping Process* (New York: McGraw-Hill, 1966).

58. Newman, J.E., and Beehr, T.A. "Personal and Organizational Strategies for Handling Job Stress: Review of Research and Opinion," *Personnel Psychology*, 32, 1977, 1–43.

59. Fuller, G.D. "Current States of Biofeedback in Clinical Practice," *American Psychologist*, 33, 1978, 39–48.

60. Lazarus, R.S. *Patterns of Adjustment* (New York: McGraw-Hill, 1976).

61. Lazarus, R.S. *Behavior Therapy and Beyond* (New York: McGraw-Hill, 1971).

62. Ibid.

63. Schein, E.H. *Career Dynamics: Matching Individual and Organizational Needs* (Reading, MA: Addison-Webb, 1978).

64. Fielding, J.E. "Worksite Health Promotion and Stress Management," *Advances*, 6, 1989, 36–40.

65. Heirich, M. "Making Stress Management Relevant to Worksite Wellness," *Advances*, 6, 1989, 55–60.

66. Jaffe, D.T.; Scott, C.D.; and Orioli, E.M. "Stress Management: Programs and Prospects," *American Journal of Health Promotion*, 84, 1986, 29–37.

67. Pelletier, K.R., and Lutz, R. "Mindbody Goes to Work: A Critical Review of Stress Management Programs in the Workplace," *Advances*, 6, 1989, 28–34.

68. Frecknall, P. Op. cit.

69. Wilson, B.R. Cardiovascular risk reduction. 46th Annual Convention of the International Council of Psychologists: East-West dialogue: The role of psychologists in promoting health and well-being. *International-Psychologist*, 29, 1989, 49–54.

70. Baun, W.B.N.; Bernacki, E.J.; and Tsai, S.P. "A Preliminary Investigation: Effect of a Corporate Fitness Program on Absenteeism and Health Care Costs," *Journal Occupational Medicine*, 28, 1986, 18–22.

71. Warshaw, L. J. Op. cit.

72. Ibid.

73. Valdes, M.R. "A Program of Stress Management in a College Setting," *Psychotherapy in Private Practice*, 6, 1988, 43–54.

74. U.S. Department of Health and Human Services. *Federal Ex-stress*.

Pilferage and Total Quality Management **6**

EMPLOYEE PILFERAGE

Pilferage is a serious problem in most healthcare organizations, including both public and private settings such as hospitals, nursing homes, clinics, pharmacies, and other various healthcare related retail environments.

There are basically two types of pilfering—that done by outsiders (non-employees), sometimes referred to as shoplifting, and pilfering done by employees. Employee pilferage may range from taking only one or two small inexpensive items such as writing materials, toilet paper rolls, or cleaning supplies, to theft of expensive merchandise such as computers. Employees can conspire with each other or conspire with outsiders (clients or delivery persons) to steal from an employer.

Causes

Some of the key reasons for employee pilferage are

- Inflation.
- Underpayment of employees.
- A high level of unemployment.
- A bad economy or employee financial troubles.
- The challenge of trying to get away with it.

- Misplaced trust. (The number of years an employee has been with the same employer does not necessarily indicate the employee's level of honesty. A dishonest employee who has been around longer has a better chance of getting away with pilferage, being familiar with the organization and the work environment.)
- Poor inventory control and supply management, which makes the employer unaware of the extent of the pilferage.
- A lack of serious consequences to the employee caught stealing.

In a small healthcare organization such as a clinic or small retail setting, employee pilferage can result in significant loss of revenue. In severe, uncontrolled cases, the employer may even be forced out of business.

Employers in healthcare organizations should not underestimate their ability to influence employees to be honest. Use of good preventive controls, stiff loss-prevention procedures, and cleverly located security devices are powerful reminders to everyone that pilferage will not be tolerated. The supervisor and the employer should also set a personal example of honesty, conscientiousness, and integrity. This is an important step in indicating to employees that dishonesty is intolerable. The organization's director or manager should follow the same loss-prevention rules that apply to everyone, such as signing for items taken from the stockroom. It is difficult, if not impossible, for a supervisor who steals from the employer to control or discipline other employees who also steal. Employees should be encouraged to report pilferage to appropriate individuals in such a way as not to create conflict with other employees.

Supervisors and employers should not feel comfortable just because their organization is located in what is regarded as a good neighborhood. This only gives a false sense of security, because employee pilferage occurs even in the best of neighborhoods and in the best of healthcare organizations.

The dishonest employees who are successful in pilfering are the ones who test the system and are convinced that they can succeed. These employees pilfer because they feel they will not be caught or that the consequences of being caught are so minor that the benefit of stealing outweighs the risk. Each time an employee successfully steals any item, that person's confidence increases and, along with it, the danger of encouraging another employee to do the same, resulting in loss of revenue to the organization. The best way to stop such employees is to keep them off balance, keep them from developing the feeling that they can beat the system. When they are caught, they should be dismissed. A dishonest employee, working alone or in collusion with others, may find ways to successfully steal from the employer no matter how theft-proof the employer attempts to make the work environment; however, the more theft-proof the organization, the less likely that dishonest employees will continue to succeed. Dishonest employees can devise ways to get away with substantial amounts of money, materials, or goods if adequate theft-control measures are not instituted. Inexperienced supervisors and employers who suspect theft should not attempt to turn detective and try to solve the crimes themselves. This might not only be dangerous but also could ruin a criminal investigation, because it is an area in which the average supervisor is an amateur.

Preventive Measures

Several measures can be used in most healthcare organizations to help reduce employee pilferage.

1. Good employee selection procedures and appropriate orientation are the first lines of defense to reduce employee pilferage. They serve as a means of screening out potentially dishonest or undesirable employees. For a nominal fee in most states, a prospective employee's driving record can be checked for pertinent violations, such as driving while under the influence of alcohol or drugs. Also, the sheriff's department, for a nominal fee will do a complete background check on prospective employees; the report will show whether the prospective employee has been convicted of any criminal offenses and, if so, the nature of the offense. The more sensitive an employee's job, the more important it is to check the employee's background prior to employment.
2. Wide-angle mirrors and one-way mirrors installed in strategic positions especially in the stockroom, provide an opportunity to observe employees for possible pilferage. They also give the potential pilferer a sense of being watched, and thus reducing the chances of pilferage.
3. A system of closed-circuit television cameras and monitors is helpful in reducing pilferage. However, these are expensive. Fake cameras and monitors that look like real ones can be effective as a deterrent to pilfering, so long as employees are unaware that they are fake. Once employees become aware that the monitors are fake, the monitors become useless toys rather than a deterrent to pilferage.
4. Electronic devices mounted at the front entrance are also helpful, especially in retail settings such as community-based pharmacies. The devices sound an alarm when an unchecked item is taken out the door.

For this to be most effective, all items must be properly sensor tagged, and every employee must leave through the front door. Otherwise, these devices must also be mounted at all employee exits. It is possible for an employee working with someone else outside the organization to beat the system, however, so employers need to be on guard. If an employee removes the tag and pretends to charge a client for the item, the client then can leave the area with the unpaid items.

5. Security audits are also helpful in reducing pilferage, as are unannounced spot checks of cash register activity and physical inventory checks.

6. Polygraph tests are sometimes used during an investigation or prior to employment to discourage pilferage. It is advisable to consult an attorney before using polygraph tests, since they are sometimes inadmissible as proof of anything.

7. Supervisors must make it clear to employees that anyone caught stealing will be dismissed and prosecuted (settling for restitution and an apology is inviting theft to continue). Maintaining a firm and tough enforcement policy that is disseminated to all employees will help reduce pilferage. The healthcare organization's policy and procedure for dealing with employee pilferage should be made an important part of employee orientation.

8. Employers should not underpay employees to such an extent that the employees feel a need to make up the difference through pilferage. Underpayment can make dishonest employees feel that they are entitled to what they are stealing.

9. Key employees should be kept informed about the activities and findings of the person in charge of security. That way, weak points in security can be strengthened without delay. If, however, a key employee is suspected of pilfering, that employee should not be informed, since it could give the employee inside information to work with.

10. The supervisor or manager should make a dependable second check of incoming ordered products to rule out the possibility of collusive theft between delivery drivers and employees who handle the receiving of merchandise.

11. All padlocks must be snapped shut on hasps when not in use to prevent the switching of locks.

12. Keys to padlocks must be controlled. Never leave the key hanging on a nail near the lock where a dishonest employee could "borrow" it and have it duplicated.

13. Trash must not be allowed to accumulate in, or be picked up from, an area near storage sites of valuable materials.

14. The supervisor or security personnel should inspect disposal locations and garbage containers at irregular intervals for the presence of saleable items, whether or not they suspect collusion between employees and outsiders. Sometimes an employee may deliberately "throw away" good merchandise with the hope of coming back to get it from the trash area later.

15. Supervisors should maintain good communication and rapport with all employees. This will help the supervisor to create a friendly atmosphere in which employees understand that their welfare is important to the success of the organization, this makes stealing less attractive.

16. The supervisor should occasionally discuss the issue of pilferage with employees, so that they know that the supervisor is aware of the problem. However, it is important not to make employees feel as if the supervisor thinks of them as dishonest. It is also important not to insult the integrity of the employees.

17. Be alert for employees passing merchandise to their friends and relatives by ringing up (or writing up) only a few of several items on a cash register (or receipt). When in doubt, check the register tape if the amount charged seems disproportionate to the quantity of merchandise sold.

18. Discourage employees from coming to work with bags or large purses. Some organizations have a policy of checking employee bags and other personal items or of requiring everyone to pass through a detection device as they leave work. If that is your organization's policy, emphasize it and follow it.

19. Do not put the cash register next to an adding machine in the checkout area, because an employee can total up sales on the adding machine, give the tape to a customer as a receipt, and keep the money because it was not registered. Insist on having every item appropriately checked out and accounted for.

20. Check the organization's duplicate carbon receipts, and cross check any duplicate receipts written in ink, when the customer should have received the original in ink. Duplicates in ink may conceal a discrepancy between the amount on the original receipt given to the customer and the duplicate, which the organization retains, especially with cash purchases.

Pilferage is a serious, expensive problem that can be better avoided with appropriate preventive measures. Be cautious when dealing with the issue of pilferage, especially be cautious when relying on someone else's findings, avoid jumping to the wrong conclusion and falsely accusing an innocent employee of pilfering. Things are sometimes not what they seem; that's why it is important to exercise caution when dealing with employee theft.

TOTAL QUALITY MANAGEMENT (TQM)

TQM Defined

Total Quality Management (TQM) is a commitment to excellence by everyone in the organization through continuous improvement—a commitment to delivering high-quality services to meet or exceed customers', clients', or consumers' expectations. The consumer is often the user of the product or services provided by healthcare providers; clients and customers are consumers. These consumers are the patients the organization serves. A client can be defined as a consumer who is not a professional and is thus unable to determine the nature of the services needed from the professional, because the client lacks the expertise to make such decisions. The client therefore heavily relies on the judgment of the professional to provide the needed services or product. For instance, the patient relies on the physician for an appropriate surgical procedure in the best interest of the patient. The patient often lacks the expertise to tell the anesthesiologist how much anesthesia to use during surgery. A customer, on the other hand, can make significant decisions about the products and services provided. For instance, a customer shopping for eyeglass frames will decide what type, style, color, and price are acceptable. Clients and customers can be primary or secondary consumers.

It is important to note that TQM addresses quality as defined or perceived by the customer, not as defined or perceived by the provider. Quality services are what the customer or client says they are. The customer's and client's needs and concerns should dominate the provider's decision making. TQM in the healthcare setting provides high-quality services to delight the client or customer. It recognizes that to do more with less, as is now demanded in healthcare, it cannot be business as usual. The goal of TQM is to meet or exceed the customer's and client's expectations with service provided in a cost-effective and efficient manner.

TQM is a people-focused management system with the purpose of continually increasing the satisfaction of consumers. One of the major assumptions of TQM is that continual organizational improvement of the workplace is always possible and necessary for an organization's optimal growth and even for survival. This may mean examining how work is accomplished and identifying how best to improve on the work for enhanced customer and client satisfaction. Other "total quality" abbreviations are TQ for Total Quality and CQI for Continuous Quality Improvement. TQM revolves around basic principles such as

- Emphasizing the primary goal of customer and client satisfaction and delight.
- Emphasizing team effort and working together by all those involved in providing services or products to the consumer.
- Preventing errors, which can reduce cost and decrease customer satisfaction. In healthcare, serious errors cost human lives, so the importance of preventing and reducing errors cannot be overemphasized.
- Developing and using data to monitoring the overall goal of delighting clients and customers.
- Stressing learning and adapting to continual change in the workplace as keys to organizational growth and survival.
- Empowering everyone in the organization to act to satisfy the consumer.
- Encouraging employee involvement, which encourages suggestions for change and trying new ideas, to delight the consumer.
- Identifying non–value-added steps and time-wasting steps to be eliminated.

Total Quality Management replaces the notion "If it is not broken, don't fix it" with "Even if it may not be broken, if it can be improved upon, then improve it." TQM stresses the power of team action for total consumer satisfaction and consumer-driven measurements.

Implementing TQM

1. Plan. The organization must identify its vision, goals, objectives, and consumers. For most healthcare organizations, the consumers are not limited to patients and others who use the organization's services or buy its products, but include intermediaries between the healthcare providers and the patients. Some of these intermediaries are called gatekeepers: health benefit managers working for insurance companies or HMOs, for example.

2. Communicate to all employees the organizational vision, goals, and objectives.
3. Identify consumers' needs and expectations from the consumers' perspective, using tools such as surveys.
4. Identify problem areas and barriers to achieving consumer satisfaction. To achieve this it is important to consider the answers to the following questions:
   - Are some problems more important than others? Why?
   - How will improvement be measured?
   - What process(es) needs to be improved?

5. Develop cross-functional teams that include managers, employees, and consumers to work on the problems and develop solutions. The team leader should encourage input from everyone.
6. Collect and analyze data on consumer satisfaction and barriers to meeting and exceeding the consumer's expectations. This will provide answers to the following questions:
   - What is/are the cause(s) of consumer's dissatisfaction?
   - Are data available to document the cause(s)?

7. Identify solutions to the identified problems:
   - What are possible solutions? (Brainstorm.)
   - Evaluate possible solutions.

8. Categorize solutions as short-range or long-range plans for implementation.
   - Pilot-test applicable solutions.
   - Evaluate the results of the pilot tests.

9. Implement the solutions and provide employee training where needed.
10. Reward employees through an appropriate reward and recognition system for goal achievement.
11. Continuously (annually) review and monitor improvements.

(For a diagram of the Total Quality Management improvement process, see figure 15.)

Basic Tools for Implementing and Monitoring TQM

Some basic statistical tools are beneficial in successfully implementing and monitoring TQM efforts. These are

Figure 15. *The Total Quality Management Improvement Process*

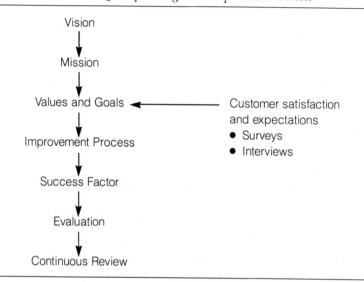

1. Data collection using surveys or questionnaires, and interviews, which can be used during planning, for customer and client identification and for problem identification and solution. Surveys are developed to serve specific needs. The survey to identify and categorize customers may be different from one assessing customer expectations and solutions to identified problems.
2. Flow charts, which are beneficial for providing a visual image of processes. For example, what steps does a patient go through from the time the patient makes an appointment to the time that patient leaves the clinic? Use of flow charts can eliminate time-wasting steps and non–value-added steps.
3. Graph include regular graphs, bar graphs, pie charts, histograms, and scatter diagrams. These can be used to plot and chart errors or consumer or client complaints by type and frequency in the healthcare organization. They can also be used for monitoring purposes, such as monthly comparative analyses of errors by type and frequency.

Sometimes attempts to implement TQM fail. Such failure has been attributed to several causes. Boyett and Conn identified 10 mistakes often made in implementing Total Quality Management.[1] These mistakes are summarized below:

1. Focusing on changing culture rather than changing the behavior of those working in the organization.
2. Failing to completely, clearly, and accurately define performance requirements and expectations.
3. Failing to develop a strategic quality plan before implementing TQM.
4. Failure to establish a functioning Executive Quality Council made up of senior managers in the organization who are responsible for successfully implementing TQM.
5. Failure to establish quality measures and goals.
6. Failure to change the compensation system to one that rewards quality leadership and results.
7. Failing to place employees physically and emotionally close to the customers and clients they serve.
8. Relying on training or quality improvement techniques as a substitute for implementing TQM. Tools are means to achieving TQM; they are not TQM by themselves. Total Quality Management is not one thing but everything done in the workplace to eliminate errors and delight the consumer.
9. Failure to provide follow-up after TQM training to ensure that learned skills are implemented in the workplace.
10. Looking for short-term breakthroughs rather than long-term, continuous improvements.

CHAPTER 6 REFERENCE

1. Boyett, Joseph H., and Conn, Henry P. "What's Wrong With Total Quality Management?" *Tapping the Network Journal*, Spring 1992, 10–14.

SUGGESTED READINGS ON TOTAL QUALITY MANAGEMENT

Berwick, Donald M.; Godfrey, A. Blanton; and Roessner, Jane. *Curing Health Care: New Strategies for Quality Improvement* (San Francisco: Jossey-Bass, 1990).

Crosby, Philip B. *Quality is Free: The Art of Making Quality Certain* (New York: McGraw-Hill, 1979).

Crosby, Philip B. *Quality Without Tears* (New York: McGraw-Hill, 1984).

Goldzimer, Linda Silverman. *"I'm First;" Your Customer's Message to You* (New York: Rawson Assoc., MacMillan, 1989).

Hauser, John R., and Clausing, Don. "The House of Quality," *Harvard Business Review*, 66, 3, 1988, 63–73.

Ishikawa, Kaoru. *What is Total Quality Control? The Japanese Way* (New York: Prentice Hall, 1985).

Johnson, H. Thomas. *Relevance Regained: From Top-Down Control to Bottom-Up Empowerment* (New York: The Free Press, 1992).

Juran, Joseph M. *Juran on Leadership for Quality: An Executive Handbook* (New York: The Free Press, 1989).

Robinson, Alan, ed., *Continuous Improvement in Operations: a Systematic Approach to Waste Reduction* (Cambridge, MA: Productivity Press, 1991).

Schein, Edgar H. *Organizational Culture and Leadership* (San Francisco: Jossey-Bass, 1985).

Schonberger, Richard J. *Building a Chain of Customers: Linking Business Functions to Create the World Class Company* (New York: The Free Press, 1990).

Roberts, Harry V., and Sergesketter, Bernard F. *Quality Is Personal: A Foundation for Total Quality Management* (New York: The Free Press, 1993).

Taguchi, Genichi, and Clausing, Don. "Robust Quality," *Harvard Business Review*, 68, 1, 1990, 65–75.

Townsend, Patrick L., with Gebhardt, Joan E. *Commit to Quality* (New York: John Wiley and Sons, 1990).

Cornesky, Robert, et al. *W. Edwards Deming: Improving Quality in Colleges and Universities* (Madison, WI: Magna Publications, Inc., 1990).

Regulatory Aspects of Personnel Management

7

EMPLOYMENT DISCRIMINATION
by Mable Smith-Pittman, R.N., Ph.D., J.D.

Introduction

Many laws provide workers with protection against discrimination in the workplace. The most significant piece of federal legislation dealing with employment discrimination is Title VII of the Civil Rights Act of 1964.[1] It prohibits employment discrimination based on race, sex, religion, or national origin, and applies to employers, employment agencies, apprenticeship programs, and labor organizations whose activities affect interstate commerce.[2] In addition to Title VII, other federal and state laws have been enacted to prohibit discrimination in the work environment. In many cases, the state and federal laws are similar, but when there is a conflict,

---

The information presented in this chapter is for general information and is not to be considered in the same light as statements of position contained in interpretative bulletins published in the *Federal Register* and the *Code of Federal Regulations*, or in the official opinion letters of the Wage and Hour Administrator or any other government agency.

federal law preempts state law. This chapter will discuss some of these laws.

The Americans With Disabilities Act (ADA)

The passage into law of the Americans With Disabilities Act (ADA)[3] in 1990 ensured that the rights of handicapped persons would be accorded appropriate legal protection. The ADA, like its predecessor, Section 504 of the Rehabilitation Act,[4] was designed to protect persons with disabilities from deprivations based on the fears, stereotypes, and prejudices of others. The Act provided clear, consistent, enforceable standards to address discriminatory practices. Under section 504, any recipient of federal funding is prohibited from discriminating on the basis of disability. Specifically, the Act provided

> No otherwise qualified handicapped individual in the United States, . . . shall, solely by reason of his handicap, be excluded from participation in, be denied the benefits of, or be subjected to discrimination under any program or activity receiving federal financial assistance . . ."[5]

Many of the terms and requirements of the ADA were derived from the Rehabilitation Act; however, the ADA greatly expanded coverage and protection against discrimination. Specific portions of the ADA cover the private sector (Title I), the activities of state and local governments (Title II), public accommodations (Title III), telecommunications services (Title IV), and a miscellaneous category (Title V).[6]

An employer is prohibited from discriminatory practices against qualified handicapped individuals in all aspects of employment practices, including job application procedures, hiring, firing, advancement, compensation, and training. A qualified individual with a disability is a person who meets legitimate skill, experience, education, or other requirements of a position and who can perform the essential functions of the position with or without reasonable accommodations.[7] The ADA, however, does not require an employer to give preference to a qualified applicant with a disability.

To establish that a violation of the ADA has occurred, a plaintiff (an employee or applicant for employment) must prove the elements of a four-pronged test.[8] First, the plaintiff must establish that he or she is a handicapped individual, defined as "any person who (i) has a physical or mental impairment which substantially limits one or more of such person's major life activities, (ii) has a record of such an impairment, or (iii) is regarded as having such an impairment." [9] Second, the individual must be otherwise qualified—defined as being able to, with or without reasonable accommodations, perform the essential functions of the position. Third, the plaintiff must be excluded from the program or denied the position solely because of handicap. Finally, the program must receive federal financial assistance.

Courts will, however, balance the responsibilities of an organization against the rights of the handicapped individual. In *Doherty* v. *Southern College of Optometry*, [10] a student's visual and neurological condition prevented him from fulfilling the clinical proficiency requirements. Doherty was successfully completing the program until new clinical requirements were added to the curriculum. The court, in addressing the "otherwise qualified" provision of the four-pronged test, noted that an individual is otherwise qualified if he is able to meet all of a program's requirements in spite of the handicap. Doherty was not otherwise qualified because his handicap prevented him from determining how much pressure he was exerting on the eyeball, thereby creating danger for prospective patients. The Southern College of Optometry had a duty to ensure that its graduates gave safe and efficient care to patients. The university was allowed the right to establish criteria for professional practice.

Similarly, courts have acknowledged that an institution or organization does not have to lower standards or make substantial alterations as part of reasonable accommodation. Reasonable accommodation is defined as "any modification or adjustment to a job or the work environment that will enable an applicant or employee with a disability to participate in the application process or to perform essential job functions." [11] Such modifications or adjustments include making existing facilities accessible to and usable by an individual with a disability, restructuring a job, modifying work schedules, modifying or acquiring equipment, and providing support personnel. [12] However, an employer is not required to make accommodations that would create an undue hardship, either financial or physical, on the operation of the business.

The case of *Wynne* v. *Tufts University School of Medicine* [13] illustrates this principle. Steven Wynne brought a discrimination action against the university alleging that he was learning disabled and that his dismissal from the School of Medicine was in violation of the Rehabilitation Act. Wynne failed 8 of 15 first-year courses. Instead of dismissing him in accordance with the school's guidelines, the dean had allowed him to repeat the first year of medical school. At the university's insistence and expense, Wynne underwent neuropsychological testing, which revealed information-processing weaknesses and cognitive deficits. Although no diagnosis of a learning disorder was made, Tufts arranged to supply Wynne with tutors, counselors, and other educational assistance. Nevertheless, Wynne still failed two of the first-year courses. Tufts then allowed Wynne to take make-up examinations in the two courses; he failed one. His request to take the examination in an altered format was denied and he was dismissed from the university. Wynne claimed that his disability placed him at a disadvantage in taking multiple-choice examinations and that Tufts University had failed to make reasonable efforts to accommodate his handicap.

The court in this instance formulated a test for determining whether an academic institution adequately meets the "reasonable accommodation" requirement.

> If the institution submits undisputed facts demonstrating that the relevant officials within the institution considered alternative means, whether the alternatives were feasible, the cost, and the effect on the academic program, and came to a rationally justifiable conclusion that the available alternatives would result either in lowering academic standards or requiring substantial program alterations, the court could rule as a matter of law that the institution had met its duty of seeking reasonable accommodation.[14]

Noting that the university had considered different methods of testing proficiency in biochemistry and had concluded that the multiple-choice format was the best method, the court ruled in favor of the university. The university's decision not to allow the student to retake the examination in a different format did not constitute failure to make reasonable accommodation.

In addition, the ADA covers individuals with certain communicable diseases, such as human immunodeficiency virus (HIV) and tuberculosis. These cases, however, usually pose additional dilemmas because of the fear and stigma associated with these diseases. The United States Supreme Court has delineated additional factors to be considered in complying with the ADA when a person has a communicable disease. These factors are (1) the nature of the risk, further defined as how the disease is transmitted; (2) the duration of the risk or how long the carrier is contagious; (3) the severity of the risk or the potential of harm to third parties; and (4) the probability that the disease will be transmitted.[15]

Although the law protects individuals who have communicable diseases, it does not mandate that institutions or organizations admit, employ, or retain individuals who pose a significant threat of harm to themselves or others. In *Doe* v. *Washington University*,[16] a third-year dental student's HIV seropositive status prevented him from performing invasive procedures. The limitations on the student's ability to perform clinical procedures prevented him from successfully completing the program. In response to the student's allegations of discrimination by the university, the court ruled that a person who poses a signficant risk of communicating an infectious disease will not be otherwise qualified for the position if reasonable accommodation would not eliminate that risk. In Doe's case, the risk of transmitting the virus was present, although minimal. The appropriateness of accommodation is decided on a case-by-case basis. The principal test is "whether the accommodation will provide an opportunity for a person with a disability to achieve the same level of performance and to enjoy benefits equal to those of an average, similarly situated person without a disability."[17]

The statute allows an employer to establish defenses against a charge of discrimination.[18] First, an employer can claim that a challenged qualification, standard, test, or selection criterion is job related and consistent with a business necessity, and that a reasonable accommodation by the employer would not enable a person who does not meet the standard to perform the job. The burden is on the employer to prove this statutory defense. Second, an employer may argue that the individual constitutes a direct threat, defined as a significant risk to the health and safety of others, that cannot be eliminated by reasonable accommodation.

The Age Discrimination in Employment Act (ADEA)

The Age Discrimination in Employment Act (ADEA)[19] protects individuals over the age of 40 from discrimination at all levels of employment. Its stated purpose is "to promote employment of older persons based on their ability rather than age; to prohibit arbitrary age discrimination in employment; and to help employers and workers find ways of meeting problems arising from the impact of age on employment."[20] The law applies to employers, labor organizations, and employment agencies. Section 623 of the statute defines each of the terms. An employer is defined as "a person engaged in an industry affecting commerce who has twenty or more employees for each working day in each of twenty or more calendar weeks in the current or preceding calendar year."[21] State and local governments are within the act's coverage; however, the federal government is excluded. A labor organization is defined as "a group in which employees participate and which exists for the purpose, in whole or in part, of dealing with employers concerning grievances, labor disputes, wages, hours, or other terms or conditions of employment." [22] An employment agency is defined as "any person regularly undertaking with or without compensation to procure employees for an employer." [23]

Major provisions of the ADEA make it illegal for an employer (1) to fail or refuse to hire, or discharge, or otherwise discriminate against any individual with respect to compensation, terms, conditions, or privileges of employment because of the individual's age; (2) to limit, segregate, or classify an employee in any way that would deprive any individual of employment opportunities or otherwise adversely affect the individual's status as an employee because of the individual's age; or (3) to reduce the wage rate of any employee in order to comply with the law.

The ADEA makes exceptions for preferential treatment based on age because of a bona fide occupational qualification reasonably necessary to the normal operation of the business, a bona fide seniority system, or for-cause discipline or discharge. [24]

A plaintiff can establish a violation of ADEA by direct evidence, establishing an inference of illegal motivation based on the McDonnell Douglas standards, or with statistical proof of a pattern of discrimination. In the case of *Buckley v. Hospital Corp. of America*, [25] the plaintiff (employee) established a prima facie case of discrimination based on direct evidence. An incoming new administrator expressed surprise at the longevity of the staff and stated at a staff meeting that he wanted to "attract younger doctors and younger nurses." Although he denied the rumor that the employment of nurses who were "fat and 40" would be terminated, the administrator confirmed his belief that the hospital needed "new blood." The plaintiff had been employed at the hospital for 10 years with favorable evaluations and promotions prior to the new administration.

Several incidents led to the plaintiff's employment termination. First, the plaintiff voiced to a physician her concern about hiring a former patient with a history of drug abuse. The admininstrator and the plaintiff's supervisor informed her that her employment would be terminated if she ever again went outside the chain of command. Following that incident, the plaintiff's supervisor on numerous occasions inquired about the plaintiff's retirement plans. The plaintiff also discovered that two other employees had been asked to report any negative comments made against the administration. The plaintiff was later involved in an incident with another employee, the facts of which are heavily disputed. Nevertheless, the administrator failed to interview witnesses whose account of the incident would have been favorable to the plaintiff.

The court noted that the administrator's statements, references to retirement, and failure to interview witnesses favorable to Buckley established direct evidence of discrimination. The burden then shifted to the defendant to rebut this direct evidence of discrimination by proving with a preponderance of evidence that the same employment decision would have been reached even in the absence of age discrimination. The defendant was unable to meet this burden.

A second method of establishing a prima facie case of age discrimination can be accomplished by satisfying the four prongs of the McDonnell Douglas standards.[26] Under this test, the plaintiff must prove that he or she (1) is a member of a protected class, defined as age 40 years or older; (2) was discharged; (3) was replaced with a person outside the protected group; and (4) was qualified to do the job. The burden of proof is then on the defendant to rebut this inference of discrimination by articulating legitimate, nondiscriminatory reasons for the employment decision. Thus, in order to prevail, the plaintiff must show that the reasons offered by the employer are a pretext for a discriminatory motive.

The plaintiff in *Williams* v. *Edward Apffels Coffee Co.*[27] successfully satisfied the four-pronged test. Williams, an elderly male, worked for 22 months as a temporary employee of the coffee company. On several occasions, he requested but was denied permanent employment. In each case, the company hired someone else. The discrimination test was satisfied by showing that (1) Williams was over 40 and thus a member of the protected class; (2) he applied for and was qualified for the positions because he had performed the jobs as a temporary employee; (3) he was not hired for the positions; and (4) the positions remained opened, although briefly, after Williams was rejected. The court noted that a plaintiff does not have to show that any discrete period of time elapsed between when he was rejected and when someone else was selected.[28]

The burden of proof then shifted to Apffels Coffee Company to articulate a legitimate, nondiscriminatory reason for the employment decision. Apffels contended that it simply hired a "more qualified" person for the position and rejected Williams because he lacked prior job-related requirements. Since this established a nondiscriminatory motive, the burden shifted back to the plaintiff to establish that the proffered reason was a pretext for discrimination. To meet this burden, Williams offered specific, detailed information on the five employees selected over him, revealing that three of the five people hired were relatives of company employees, two had no experience, and two had limited experience. Ruling for the plaintiff, the court held that a genuine issue of fact existed as to whether the employer's alleged reason for not hiring Williams was a pretext for a discriminatory motive.

The ADEA makes exceptions for preferential treatment based on age. An employer may make unfavorable employment decisions if reasonable non–age-related factors are used. The defendant must present evidence of a legitimate nondiscriminatory reason of sufficient clarity and rationality. In *Houser* v. *Sears*,[29] the court reversed a jury's verdict in favor of the plaintiff whose employment was terminated after a deliberate misapplication of funds from one customer's account to another.

Another defense against a charge of ADEA violation is the bona fide occupational qualification exception. The burden is on the defendant employer to establish that (1) the age limit is reasonably necessary to the essence of the business; (2) all or substantially all individuals excluded from the job involved are in fact disqualified; or (3) some of the individuals so excluded possess a disqualifying trait that cannot be ascertained except by reference to age.[30]

Sex Discrimination

Sex discrimination is prohibited by Title VII, by the Equal Pay Act (EPA), by Executive Order 11246, by various federal laws governing receipt of federal financial assistance, and by state laws.[31] Under Title VII, it is unlawful for an employer to refuse to hire; to discharge; or to otherwise discriminate against, limit, segregate, or classify employees on the basis of sex. This prohibition also applies to labor unions and employment agencies.

Employers are prohibited from asking questions of female applicants that are not asked of male applicants. Examples of practices that violate Title VII include asking only female applicants about pregnancy and child care plans. In *Bruno* v. *City of Crown Point*,[32] the court noted that an "employer is not required to ignore an applicant's family and family responsibilities." However, the questions must be asked in a neutral, nondiscriminatory manner of all applicants, regardless of sex. The court in *Barbano* v. *Madison County*[33] found that an employer's asking a female applicant whether her "husband would object to her running around the country with men" and making comments that "he did not want to hire a woman who would get pregnant and quit" were sexually discriminatory.

Title VII makes exceptions for sex discrimation if sex is a bona fide occupational qualification (BFOQ) reasonably necessary to the normal operation of that particular business or enterprise. Sedmak and Vidas identified four categories in which employers have raised the BFOQ exception: (1) ability to perform; (2) same-sex, personal contact; (3) customer preference; and (4) pregnancy or fetal protection.[34] The "ability to perform" exception is raised when an employer bars a female from certain jobs based on the assumption that she is physically or mentally unable to handle the job responsibilities. The guiding principle is that employment practices barring women from certain jobs based on invalid information or invalid beliefs of their inability to perform usually violate Title VII.[35] Similarly, employers cannot use pregnancy and fetal concerns to justify a BFOQ exception.[36]

Although the preference of customers is not a BFOQ exception, the needs of an organization can necessitate a gender-based policy. The *Moteles*[37] court ruled that the university's policy of rotating females to different shifts to ensure that a female officer was available to handle sexual assault cases was a BFOQ exception. In contrast, the court in *In Re Pan American World Airlines, Inc.*[38] rejected the airline's contention that a gender-based policy was necessary to ensure passenger safety and therefore was a BFOQ exception. The airline had a maternity leave policy that required a pregnant flight attendant to notify them of the pregnancy and to take leave without pay until 60 days after the birth, at which time the attendant would return to work.

The Family and Medical Leave Act (FMLA)

The passage into law of the Family and Medical Leave Act (FMLA)[39] was designed to ensure that parents are able to participate in early childrearing and that men and women can partipate in caretaking activities for ill family members without having to choose between the job and family responsibilities. Its stated purposes are

1) to balance the demands of the workplace with the needs of families, to promote the stability and economic security of families, and to promote national interests in preserving family integrity;
2) to entitle employees to take reasonable leave for medical reasons, for the birth or adoption of a child, and for the care of a child, spouse, or parent who has a serious health condition;

3) to accomplish the purpose described in paragraphs (1) and (2) in a manner that accommodates the legitimate interests of employers;

4) to accomplish the purpose described in paragraphs (1) and (2) in a manner that, consistent with the Equal Protection Clause of the Fourteenth Amendment, minimizes the potential for employment discrimination on the basis of sex by ensuring generally that leave is available for eligible medical reasons (including maternity-related disability) and for compelling family reasons, on a gender-neutral basis; and

5) to promote the goal of equal employment opportunity for women and men, pursuant to such clause.[40]

FMLA requires employers with 50 or more employees to provide up to 12 weeks of leave during any 12-month period. An eligible employee is one who has been employed "for at least 12 months by the employer with respect to whom leave is requested under section 2612 of this title; and for at least 1,250 hours of service with such employer during the previous 12-month period."[41] The act authorizes leave for (1) birth, adoption, foster care, or care of a child; (2) care of a spouse, parent, or child with a serious health condition; or (3) a serious health condition that renders the employee unable to work.[42] "Serious health condition" means an illness, injury, impairment, or physical or mental condition that involves inpatient care in an acute-care center, hospital, or residential medical care facility, or continuous treatment by a healthcare provider.[43] Voluntary or cosmetic treatments that are not considered serious may not be protected by the FMLA; routine preventive examinations are excluded as well.

All reasonable efforts must be made to comply with the FMLA and to create a smooth leave transition. Employers and employees both have responsibilities under the FMLA. Employers are prohibited from discriminating against employees who take leave under the FMLA. However, an employer can require that an employee's request for leave be supported by "a certification issued by the health care provider of the eligible employee or of the son, daughter, spouse, or parent of the employee, as appropriate."[44] The employee must provide the employer with at least 30 days' notice if the leave is foreseeable, as soon as is practicable if it is not foreseeable.[45] In addition, the employee must comply with the employer's request for certification in a timely manner. The employee should consult with the employer and indicate whether leave will be taken intermittently or on a reduced work schedule.

The National Labor Relations Act (NLRA) or Wagner Act

A significant piece of federal law that regulates the employer-employee relationship is the National Labor Relations Act (NLRA).[46] The right of employees to engage in collective bargaining activities was established in 1935 with the passage of the NLRA, also known as the Wagner Act. Designed to promote unionization in a bureaucratic, industrial workplace, the NLRA has undergone several modifications, including the Taft-Hartley amendments in 1947 and the Health Care amendments in 1974. The Taft-Hartley amendments were in response to the United States Supreme Court's decision in *Packard Motor Car Co.* v. *NLRB*[47] that the wording of the act did not exclude supervisory personnel from the act's protection. These amendments removed supervisors from collective bargaining protection in an effort to equalize the balance of power between management and workers.

The National Labor Relations Board (NLRB) is the administrative agency entrusted with enforcing the act. Its basic scope is to determine the outcome of an election, oversee elections of collective bargaining units, and investigate claims of unfair labor practices.

Because the intent of the NLRA is to promote a peaceful bargaining process, both the employer and employee have responsibilities. Section 8(a)(2) of the NLRA makes it an unfair labor practice for an employer to "dominate or interfere with the formation or administration of any labor organization or contribute financial or other support to it . . ."[48] Employers must also bargain in good faith with the intent to negotiate or settle disputes. Employees, on the other hand, are prohibited from engaging in collective bargaining activities during working hours. They also have the right to strike; however, employers must be given advance notice. A strike is defined as a collective quitting of work to induce the employer to agree to the demands of the union representative. Fair labor practices prohibit employers from terminating the employment of striking workers; however, management may hire replacement workers to continue business operations. The act prevents unlawful discrimination against employees for their participation in union activities.

The case of *Waterbury Hospital* v. *N.L.R.B.*[49] discussed the rights of employers and unions during and after a strike. In *Waterbury*, a nonprofit community hospital with a nursing staff of 600 failed to reach an agreement with the union. In response to the resulting strike, the hospital shut down. Several weeks later, the hospital reopened several of its units, staffing them with managerial and supervisory nurse employees, crossover nurses (nurses who abandoned the strike), and newly hired nurses. The hospital guaranteed the latter two groups their preferred positions and shifts. Four months later, despite disagreements between the hospital and union regarding the treatment of striking nurses, a new collective bargaining agreement was reached.

The union, however, continued to pursue a claim of unfair labor practice against the hospital for its position that striking nurses would not be guaranteed their prestrike positions and that nonstrikers would not be "bumped" from their chosen positions for at least 12 months. The hospital contended that they were forced during the strike to hire new nurses as permanent employees to maintain some business operations. The board found and the court affirmed that the hospital had committed unfair labor practices, on the basis that some nonstrikers had been given poststrike positions that they had not occupied during the strike. In some cases, the nonstrikers were given preference for positions in departments that had been closed during the strike.

WORKERS' COMPENSATION
by Mable Smith-Pittman, R.N., Ph.D., J.D., and Eucharia E. Nnadi, Ph.D., J.D.

If an employee is injured or gets sick because of work conditions, the employee may be entitled to benefits for all resulting medical costs. If that injury or illness causes a disability for several days or if the employee is permanently impaired, he or she may also be entitled to partial payment of lost wages. The workers' compensation program is therefore an insurance plan provided by the employer; it pays all costs for medically necessary services if an employee is injured or becomes sick because of work conditions.

Employers who have three or more employees may be required to have workers' compensation insurance. A contractor who sublets any part of a contract to a subcontractor may be liable for any employees of the subcontractor not covered through an insurance company or through a self-insurance program approved by the state division of workers' compensation. The insurance coverage must be provided by the employer for all employees at no cost to them.

Advantages of Workers' Compensation Programs

There are several advantages of workers' compensation insurance:

- In the case of an employee's injury or death on the job, the employer is protected against any suit by the employee, the employee's legal representative, spouse, or anyone otherwise entitled to recover damages from the employer on account of such injury or death.
- The employer knows in advance just how much the coverage will cost and can budget this expense throughout the year.
- Carrying workers' compensation insurance reduces costly litigation and provides a comparatively speedy, simple, and inexpensive procedure for payment of compensation, regardless of who is at fault.
- Workers' compensation is intended to be a fair means of determining compensation, based on wages paid and the extent of the injury.
- Immediate medical treatment is provided to the injured employee for as long as it is needed.
- An owner or partner working full time in a business may elect to be covered under workers' compensation.
- Workers' compensation provides reasonable assurance that injured workers will be cared for.

Although an exempt or excluded employer is not required to secure the payment of compensation to excluded employees, the employer may voluntarily waive the exclusion. By taking out a workers' compensation policy, the employer can secure for the employees the benefits of the workers' compensation law and secure for the employer the protection and advantages of the law.

An employer, once notified of a violation of the law, may be enjoined from conducting business until payment of compensation has been secured. In addition, any employer who fails to secure such compensation can be charged and, upon conviction, will be punished for violation.

Although state requirements vary, there are generally three ways to comply with the law:

1. An employer may obtain a workers' compensation insurance policy through an insurance agency.
2. The employer may qualify as a self-insurer by submitting an application and fulfilling the financial bonding and excess liability insurance re-

quirements by showing the required financial net worth and by fulfilling other requirements as determined by the state.

3. The employer may join a self-insurers' fund sponsored by an association of which the employer is a member.

Most employers comply by purchasing a workers' compensation policy from an insurance company of their choice.

Qualifying Employees

The definition of qualifying employees differs from state to state; however, the information provided below, in general, applies to most states. It is prudent to check your particular state law.

In determining employer liability, part-time workers count as employees, as do student workers and any members of the employer's family employed full or part time. Individual owners or partners are not counted as employees; however, if they work full time in the business and give prior notice to the state division of workers' compensation they may elect to be covered under the insurance policy issued to their company.

Any corporate officer who performs services for remuneration for the corporation, whether full time or part time, is considered an employee. Any corporate officer, by giving notice to the state division of workers' compensation, may by exempt from coverage.

"Casual" employees are counted as employees and are entitled to the benefits of the law, unless their employment is both casual and not "in the course" of the trade, business, profession, or occupation of the employer. Maintenance, repair, painting, cleaning, and the like are in the course of business because the business could not carry on without them and because they are an expected, routine, and inherent part of carrying on any enterprise.

Under the workers' compensation law, the employee usually has a right to

1. A safe working place.
2. Insurance protection in case of a job-related injury or illness, beginning with the first day on the job.
3. Prompt payment of benefits provided by the law.
4. Periodic reports from the division of workers' compensation, the insurance company, and the employer on the status of any claim.
5. Copies of any medical reports requested by the employer.

6. Assistance from the division of workers' compensation, including complete information about the workers' compensation law.

In order to receive workers' compensation benefits, the employee generally has to

1. Promptly report job-related injury or illness to the employer.
2. Use the doctor chosen by the employer or by the employer's insurance company. If the employee is not satisfied with that doctor, the employer or insurance carrier may select a different one.
3. Cooperate with any rehabilitation program considered necessary to help the employee return to work.
4. Report, on request, any earnings, including Social Security benefits and unemployment compensation benefits.
5. Provide the employer's insurance company with all receipts for medical costs paid that relate to a workers' compensation case. This is necessary before an employee can be reimbursed for the medical costs paid that are covered by workers' compensation insurance.

Medical Benefits

Workers' compensation will generally pay the following costs resulting from a job-related injury or illness:

1. Medical, surgical, or hospital care.
2. Prescribed items, such as drugs, braces, prosthetic devices, and wheelchairs.
3. Rehabilitation and training in preparation for the employee's return to work (in cases of severe injury).
4. Reasonable travel costs associated with going to and from the doctor or hospital. Reimbursement is usually available only for travel necessary for treatment, not for such trips as visits to the drugstore.

Rehabilitation Benefits

Rehabilitation services for injured workers who need help to return to their jobs usually include

1. Counseling and guidance.
2. Assistance from rehabilitation nurses with medication, nursing consultation, nutrition, personal hygiene instruction, and home modification for the severely injured.

3. Transportation arrangements for doctor visits and other necessary travel.
4. Vocational testing and evaluation for persons who need special training before they can return to work.
5. On-the-job training or vocational training for people who need additional skills to return to work.
6. Assistance with the use, care, and replacement of prosthetic devices.
7. Monitoring of rehabilitation services provided by any approved rehabilitation service provider.

Cash Benefits

If an employee cannot work because of a job-related injury or illness, and if the injury or illness causes disability for the number of days specified by law, the employee is entitled to payments to replace part of the lost wages. The amount of money an employee receives depends on (1) the employee's average weekly wage at the time of injury or becoming ill; (2) the severity of disability; and (3) whether the employee receives other benefits, such as unemployment compensation or Social Security payments. The division of workers' compensation can help determine the amount of payments an employee should receive.

Types of Disability

1. Temporary Total disability prevents an employee from working during a limited period of time.
2. Temporary Partial disability allows an employee to work in a limited capacity during recovery. Compensation for this type of disability is often not automatic. The employer's insurance company usually sends appropriate forms for the employee to use to request payment for wage loss.
3. Permanent Impairment results in amputation, loss of a significant percentage of vision in either eye after correction, or serious facial or head disfigurement. Compensation is based on a rating that follows American Medical Association guidelines after the employee has reached maximum improvement (when the employee has recovered as much as can be expected).
4. Permanent Total disability prevents the employee from returning to work.

If an employee receives Social Security disability payments and workers' compensation benefits, the latter may be reduced so that the two combined will not exceed a certain percentage of what the employee was earning before being injured.

5. Death benefits are payable to surviving dependents of a worker who dies because of a job-related accident or illness. The amount will vary according to the number of dependents, and from state to state. There is usually a maximum amount paid, and a limited amount of burial costs may also be paid. If there are no dependents, compensation may not be paid, except for burial costs.

The basic theory behind all workers' compensation programs is that an employee should be compensated for work-related injury without the need for expensive and lengthy litigation. It is a no-fault system; the employee does not have to prove employer negligence in order to prevail. The trade-off is that workers' compensation is the exclusive remedy for employees or their dependents against employers for employment-related injuries or diseases. Therefore, the employer is ideally immune from nonintentional tort lawsuits.

The Federal Employees Compensation Act (FECA)[50] provides coverage for federal employees and their dependents for personal injury, disability, or death sustained in the performance of duty. Under the federal system, the Secretary of Labor supervises administrative claims through the Office of Workers' Compensation Programs.[51]

State workers' compensation statutes differ in a variety of ways, but maintain the common theme that an employee is entitled to certain benefits for a personal injury or death arising out of and in the course of employment. This coverage formula has three components that are often the basis of extensive litigation. First, workers' compensation coverage is limited to employees, as opposed to volunteers or independent contractors. In deciding whether an individual is an employee, courts will look at the nature of the work rendered, the scope and purpose of the work activities, the duration and regularity of service, the nature of payment, and any agreements between the parties.

The coverage formula also contains the "arising out of" component, which looks at the extent and scope of the risk. Key questions in addressing this component include "Did the work environment increase or enhance the risks of injury, disease, or death?" "Was the risk associated with the work environment?" "Did the work environment expose the employee to the risk?" "Did the employment cause the injury?" The general rule is that an injury is compensable if the injured employee was performing a work-related activity or was put at risk by the nature of the work.

The final component in the coverage formula is the provision that the injury must take place "in the course of employment." This component looks at the relationship between the employment and the injury—specifically, the time, place, and circumstances as they relate to employment.[52] "Is there a connection between the time and place of the injury and the requirements of employment?" is the key question. Litigation issues center around whether or not the employee, at the time of injury, was acting within the scope of employment or had so deviated from the scope of employment as to have abandoned employment activities. As a general rule, an employee is not covered under workers' compensation for injuries sustained while traveling to and from work. This includes injuries sustained while in the employer's parking lot. In *Sentara Leigh Hosp. v. Nichols*,[53] the Virginia Court of Appeals denied workers' compensation benefits to a home health nurse who was injured while driving from her home to a patient's home. The court noted that the nature of the nurse's employment required her to visit patients, therefore the "coming and going" rule barred compensation. Because exceptions to the general rules are made and because each case is decided based on its facts, it is difficult to speculate as to case outcomes. The case of *Peterson v. W.C.A.B.*[54] illustrates this principle. The court addressed several exceptions to the general rule that an injury sustained while an employee is going to or coming from work does not occur in the course of employment and is therefore not covered under workers' compensation. The exceptions are

1. The claimant's employment contract includes transportation to and from work.
2. The claimant has no fixed place of work.
3. The claimant is on a special mission for the employer.
4. Special circumstances apply such that the claimant was furthering the business of the employer.

The clamaint worked as a nurse for a temporary agency, whose principal business was supplying healthcare providers to various healthcare facilities on an as-needed basis. The agency would contact the provider with an assignment and pay the provider on a hourly rate from the time of signing into the assigned facility. No expenses were paid for travel time or for mileage. Ruling for the claimant, the court addressed two exceptions to the general rule. First, a nurse employed by a temporary agency does not have a fixed place of employment. Second, the nurse was furthering the business of the employer when she traveled to the assigned workplace.

Each state statute will identify the agency that has jurisdiction over workers' compensation claims. The state agency can usually hear disputed claims and perform those duties that have been conferred by statute. Certain provisions of workers' compensation claims are constantly repealed and amended; therefore, a review of the state's workers' compensation statue is the initial starting point.

EMPLOYMENT AT WILL
by Mable Smith-Pittman, R.N., Ph.D., J.D.

The "employment at will" doctrine provides that the employment relationship may be terminated at the will of either the employer or the employee without further obligations. This doctrine is in contrast with employment relationships based on a formal legal employment contract, which severely limits the employer's ability to terminate employment. Any employee who does not have an employment contract is classified as an at-will employee and can be dismissed at any time with or without cause. Recently, because of the harshness of this doctrine, there has been a "trend toward a restricted application of the at-will employment rule whereby the right of an employer to discharge an at-will employee without cause is limited by either public policy considerations or an implied covenant of good faith and fair dealing." [55]

In the absence of an implied or expressed contract, a dismissed at-will employee can establish a case of wrongful discharge by alleging one or both exceptions to the at-will doctrine. The "public policy" exception provides that employment may not be terminated for reasons that are inconsistent with public policy, such as discrimination, whistle blowing, refusing to commit a moral or legal wrong, or filing a workers' compensation claim. This exception is based on the theory that a person should act in the best interests of society and to protect the public at large.

An employer has an obligation to treat an at-will employee with fairness and to maintain a good-faith employment relationship. For example, an employer may not terminate employment simply to deprive an employee of earned compensation, such as commissions, retirement benefits, or insurance coverage. Although an employment relationship based on the "implied covenant of good faith and fair dealing" is legally not as strong as a formal contract, it provides at-will employees with some protection by subjecting bad-faith employment termination to the scrutiny of the courts.

The case of *Laudenslager v. Loral*[56] illustrates public policy exceptions to the at-will doctrine. The Chesapeake Circuit Court judge ruled that an employee who was dismissed for refusing to participate in racial discrimination could bring an action for wrongful discharge. In addition, the court interpreted the at-will doctrine to require "each party to an employment relationship to give the other reasonable notice of termination, unless there is an agreement or understanding to the contrary."[57] The failure to do so can be actionable as a breach of an implied contract.

An employee handbook can create enforceable contractual rights for at-will employees if the traditional contract elements are present. The *Duldulao*[58] court identified these elements:

First, the language of the policy statement must contain a promise clear enough that an employee would reasonably believe that an offer has been made. Second, the statement must be disseminated to the employee in such a manner that the employee is aware of its contents and reasonably believes it to be an offer. Third, the employee must accept the offer by commencing or continuing to work after learning of the policy statement. When these conditions are present, then the employee's continued work constitutes consideration for the promises contained in the statement, and under traditional principles a valid contract is formed.[59]

In *Daymon v. Hardin County General Hospital*,[60] the plaintiff, a nurse, was given written notice of termination for leaving her workstation without a bona fide reason. The employee handbook stated that the failure of an employee to be at the assigned job punctually or to remain on the job until quitting time was a basis for automatic dismissal. The plaintiff contended that her discharge was without cause and in violation of the policies and procedures in the employee handbook. Rejecting the breach-of-contract claim, the court ruled that the language of the employee handbook did not fulfill the first element of contract formation.

ALTERNATIVE DISPUTE RESOLUTIONS
by Mable Smith-Pittman, R.N., Ph.D., J.D.

In some jurisdictions, it takes months or years to get a lawsuit resolved, resulting in tremendous financial and emotional costs. Many of these cases could be settled outside the courtroom using alternatives to litigation. Alternative dispute resolution processes involve using outside assistance to negotiate a settlement as an alternative to litigating complaints in the court system. Two of these alternatives are mediation and arbitration.

Mediation

Mediation is a process whereby a neutral third party, known as a mediator, attempts to arrange a settlement between the parties to a complaint or lawsuit.[61] The primary responsibility for negotiating a settlement remains with the parties; the mediator's role is to assist the process. This can be accomplished by helping the parties delineate common areas of agreement, focusing areas of disagreement, offering alternatives, supervising the discussions, and drafting a settlement agreement.

The process is usually private and confidential to ensure that the parties will divulge whatever information is needed to resolve the issue. Although no two mediation sessions are identical, a common scheme is that the parties are introduced to the process, ground rules are established and agreed on, issues are identified, options are discussed, and an agreement is negotiated.[62] This allows the parties to approach the process with an attitude of problem solving and the feeling that they have input into the process.

Mediation has been used successfully in marriage dissolution, custody battles, disputes between doctors, contract disputes, and disputes between healthcare providers and healthcare facilities. Knight[63] describes how mediation was used to prevent an expensive trial over damages in a medical malpractice case. A hospital, an anesthesiologist, and an obstetrician were sued for malpractice in a brain-damage case. The hospital's lawyer wanted to settle the case, but felt that it would be difficult to apportion the damages between the two physicians. Compounding the problem was that the judge had given the attorney one hour to decide the apportionment issue before he impaneled a jury and started the trial. Mediation provided an alternative to resolve the settlement issue. The lawyers "were able to meet several times to determine the total amount of the settlement, its structure, and the apportionment of liability."[64]

Although mediation provides an alternative to the time-consuming and expensive litigation process, it is not suitable for resolving every dispute. Some parties may feel pressured into a settlement. It is important at the initiation of mediation that the parties understand the tremendous amount of control they have over the process. The parties can also decide that a settlement is not possible and even reject a previously agreed-on settlement. In other cases, mediation may not work because the parties are firm on their positions and simply want their day in court. Mediation is usually successful when the parties' goal is to resolve the dispute quickly.

Arbitration

Like mediation, arbitration offers an alternative to lengthy, expensive litigation. Arbitration is the process by which parties to a dispute voluntarily agree to submit their differences to an arbitrator for resolution. The parties can agree to arbitration before any dispute arises, as in contract clauses, or after the dispute has arisen. The involved parties select a neutral third party or a panel of individuals with knowledge of the subject matter who will hear the case and render a decision.

Arbitration is primarily used to resolve disputes over the interpretation or performance of contracts and in labor-management issues.[65] Unlike mediation, in arbitration the parties surrender control of the outcome to the arbitrator. Although the arbitrator decides the issues, the parties retain considerable control over the standards and procedures used to resolve the dispute, including whether or not the decision will be advisory or binding. Many of the details of arbitration are outlined in the arbitration clause of a contract or by a contract drafted after a dispute has arisen.

Since arbitration is a private, confidential process, there is no generalizable common scheme. However, there are several steps that must be followed. First, a party must file a demand for arbitration, which states the dispute and requests a remedy. Second, the other party replies to the demand in writing. It is conceivable that the dispute can be resolved at this stage. If not, the parties must then agree on an arbitrator or arbitration panel. An arbitration hearing is similar to a trial, in that it is a fact-finding process in which each side can examine and cross-examine witnesses. In essence, the parties try to make persuasive arguments in favor of their positions. Following the hearing, a decision is usually rendered within a previously agreed-upon time frame.

SEXUAL HARASSMENT
by Maxine Agazie, Ph.D., ACSW

Introduction

This topic defines and examines some of the troubling aspects of sexual harassment and how to prevent it in healthcare settings. It also explores the need for educational groups to be conducted in healthcare environments to reduce or eliminate sexual harassment in the workplace. Several exercises and case samples are included to assist the medical social worker in conducting educational groups designed to reduce sexual harassment in various healthcare settings. These educational groups will be didactic and interventive in nature. There are numerous advantages to be derived from conducting educational groups in healthcare settings. A group provides an excellent setting for social modeling and gives participants a chance to discuss and receive feedback from other members. A bibliography on sexual harassment is also included to help individuals as they prepare to conduct the educational groups.

Because of their professional training in facilitating educational group interactions as well as other types of groups, medical social workers are highly qualified to conduct the educational groups. Medical social workers are a vital part of the healthcare team. They are employed in hospitals, health departments, public health agencies, home healthcare services, nursing homes, inner-city clinics, and other healthcare settings.

Definitions

It is important to differentiate sex discrimination from sexual harassment. Both are unlawful practices, but they are different.

Sex discrimination is discrimination in selection, promotion, placement, or terms or conditions of employment on the basis of gender. "It shall be an unlawful employment practice for an employer . . . to fail or refuse to hire or to discharge any individual, or otherwise to discriminate against any individual with respect to his compensation, terms, conditions or privileges of employment, because of such individual's race, color, religion, *sex* or national origin" (Section 703 of Title VII of the Civil Rights Act of 1964, emphasis added).

EEOC guidelines[66] "define sexual harassment as unwelcome sexual advances, requests for sexual favors, or other verbal or physical conduct of a sexual nature when

- Submission to such conduct is made either explicitly or implicitly a term or condition of an individual's employment.
- Submission to or rejection of such conduct by an individual is used as the basis for employment decisions affecting such individuals.
- Such conduct has the purpose or effect of substantially interfering with an individual's work performance or creating an intimidating, hostile, or offensive working environment.

There are several definitions of sexual harassment. Sexual harassment has operational perspectives and may be interpreted differently by persons in the same work environment.

Goodner and Kolenich (1993)[67] agreed that the definition of sexual harassment and its legal meaning still have an element of confusion surrounding them. According to Childers-Hermann (1993),[68] sexual harassment as an official term came about in 1975.

Zuffoletto (1992)[69] suggested that there are two types of sexual harassment: quid pro quo harassment and a hostile working environment. An example of quid pro quo harassment would be a situation in which Jane Doe is seeking promotion and a pay raise, but to get them she must render sexual favors to her supervisor. An example of a hostile working environment would be that Jane Doe's place of employment has workers telling jokes that are sexually offensive and displaying sexually offensive behavior that results in Jane's not being able to perform her work duties. Margolis (1994)[70] concurred with Zuffoletto,[69] placing sexual harassment into two categories: quid pro quo harassment and a hostile working environment. She pointed out that a sexual harassment claim of a hostile working environment may be more challenging to sustain than that of quid pro quo harassment. Kinard et al.[71] (1995) agreed with Margolis[70] that a hostile environment tends to be more difficult to prove because of its subjective nature. A survey conducted in Los Angeles County reported the startling results that 67 percent of the male subjects surveyed stated that they would be flattered to be propositioned by a member of the opposite sex; 63 percent of the female subjects participating in the same survey said they would be offended if they were propositioned by a member of the opposite sex. Examples of sexual harassment in a form of a hostile work environment include but are not limited to sexual jokes; pornographic magazines in the workplace; sexually explicit oral or written messages or comments, faxes, calendars, or posters in the workplace; questions about an individual's sexual activity; and unwelcome sexual touching.

Wolfe (1996)[72] defined sexual harassment as a violation of Title VII of the Civil Rights Act. McGrath (1994)[73] of Newfoundland, who focused on women in the workplace, defined sexual harassment as sexual coercion and a poisoned work environment. Gray (1994)[74] conducted research at Georgia State University and has worked to help nursing students identify sexual harassment. In her research, she defined sexual harassment as overt or physical behavior. Sexual harassment therefore can encompass different unwelcome acts with sexual overtones that may be visual, verbal, or physical, and may include pictures or graffiti.

Reducing and Eliminating Sexual Harassment

There is a great need to reduce or eliminate sexual harassment in the workplace. According to Kinard et al. (1995),[71] a survey conducted in 1994 showed an exorbitant increase in formal charges of sexual harassment being made in healthcare settings. Nurses filed the largest numbers of complaints, according to Kinard's findings. Sexual harassment is destructive to the individual being harassed and the organization.

Another reason for the crucial need for educational groups in healthcare settings to reduce or eliminate sexual harassment is the litigious society of the 1990s. Large sums of money can be paid as damage awards to an employee who is a victim of sexual harassment. Goodner and Kolenich (1993)[67] indicated that sexual harassment contributes not only to high legal costs but also causes excessive employee turnover, poor patient care, and lost productivity on the job.

Healthcare institutions can no longer stand idly by or merely react to sexual harassment. Appropriate policy is crucial, but most of all, employees must be aware of and understand their organization's policy regarding sexual harassment. Often, sexual harassment in the workplace goes unreported because employees are afraid of retaliation.

Knowledge is a vital tool in the fight against sexual harassment. Some victims of sexual harassment in healthcare settings allow abuse to continue because they do not know what to do. They may feel inferior to the person who is sexually harassing them and may be afraid of losing their jobs if they reveal what is happening to them, or they may fear being reprimanded or further demeaned by a powerful supervisor. Men who are victims of sexual harassment by women may feel that coworkers will ridicule and laugh at them if the harassment is revealed. By educating these victims, we will empower them to handle these situations in a more constructive manner (Childers-Hermann, 1993).[68]

Feelings of apathy persist among employees who are sexually harassed. These employees may be intimidated by the power of the harasser and feel as though it would be a waste of time to file a claim of sexual harassment against such a powerful figure. Such employees should be educated about the policy and laws regarding sexual harassment. A new concept defined by the courts in 1991 is known as the "reasonable woman" standard. It further protects women because women may object to sexual statements that may not offend many men (Kinard et al., 1995).[71]

It is important to note that there can be a case of sexual harassment even if a supervisor does not directly require sexual favors from an employee in order for the employee to receive a benefit; all that may be needed is for the employee to perceive the supervisor's conduct as abusive (Williams, 1994).[75] Therefore, even though a harasser may be unaware that his or her speech or behavior constitutes sexual harassment, the harassment is unlawful and may still humiliate or intimidate the victim. Sexual harassment is often viewed from the perspective of the individual being harassed, not that of the harasser. Haratani et al. (1993)[76] concluded their paper by simply viewing sexual harassment as legally and morally wrong.

Supervisors' Responsibilities in Reducing and Eliminating Sexual Harassment

1. Develop and enforce a clear policy that sexual harassment is unlawful and will not be tolerated in the workplace.
2. Develop a work environment free of sexually oriented comments, pictures, behavior, calendars, and messages.
3. Encourage employees to report sexual harassment.
4. Investigate all reported sexual harassment cases, treat them seriously, and resolve them effectively. Ignoring sexual harassment will only make matters worse.
5. Identify and deal with potential problems as a preventive measure.
6. Conduct, or encourage others to conduct, educational groups or workshops on eliminating sexual harassment in the workplace.

Below are several tips for conducting effective educational groups at work to eliminate sexual harassment. Also included are sample case exercises for use during educational group sessions.

20 Pertinent Tips To Be Included in Educational Groups

1. Aggressively develop a written policy regarding sexual harassment in the workplace. Actively create a workplace free of sexual harassment.

2. Make it mandatory for all employees to attend educational groups conducted by the employer for the benefit of employees.
3. Discourage employees from telling lewd jokes or making sexual remarks in the workplace. Explain that what may appear to be an innocent joke may be very offensive and distasteful to another person, and thus may constitute sexual harassment.
4. Explain to healthcare workers participating in the group settings that the most crucial aspect of sexual harassment is the unwelcome sexual comments that will prevent employees from performing their work duty.
5. Explain to participants the difference between the "reasonable woman" standard and a "reasonable person" standard. Discuss the implications for sexual harassment cases.
6. Explain to healthcare supervisors and administrators that employers as well as employees can be sued for sexual harassment.
7. Discuss and give examples of the following court cases dealing with pertinent aspects of sexual harassment:
   Kopp v. *Samaritan Health System, Inc.* No. 93-1519 SI, 19193 U.S. APP LEXIS 33452.
   Harris v. *Forklift Systems, Inc.* 114 S. Ct. 367 (1993).
   Saville v. *Houston County Healthcare Authority*, 8a52 F. Supp. 1512 (M.D. Ala. 1994).
   Katz v. *Dole* (709 F2d 25 14th Cir 1983).
   Henson v. *City of Dundee* (682 F2d 897 11th Cir 1982).
   Meritor Savings Bank v. *Vinson* (477 U. S. 57(9) LED2d 49, 106, S Ct 2399, 1986).
   Ellison v. *Brady* (924 F2d 872, 1991).
8. Emphasize that historically, sexual harassment has been around since Florence Nightingales' time but it has been declared illegal since Title VII of the 1964 Civil Rights Act was created.
9. Educate the healthcare participants on verbal, nonverbal, and physical sexual harassment.
10. Make participants aware that keeping silent on the issue of sexual harassment will not make it disappear.
11. Point out that men can also be victims of sexual harassment and that they are protected under Title VII of the Civil Rights Act.
12. Remember that placing a policy regarding sexual harassment in a manual and giving it to employees is not enough to ensure that they comprehend the policy.

13. Explain the meaning of third-party liability for employers.
14. Recall that anyone accused of sexual harassment still has a right to due process.
15. Note that healthcare administrators must frequently evaluate the sexual harassment policy implemented in educational groups.
16. Consider that the medical social worker or other appropriate individual must conduct educational groups on a level that can be understood by all participating employees.
17. Construct an evaluation tool to be administered at the end of each educational group to test how much information participants obtained.
18. After providing employees with the policy manual regarding sexual harassment, have employees sign a statement saying they received the manual.
19. Discourage employees from making false charges of sexual harassment.
20. Remember that, because of differences in work settings, how often institutions need to offer educational groups on sexual harassment may vary. It is recommended to conduct groups more frequently than once a year.

Sample Exercises and Cases for Educational Group Sessions and Workshops

The following exercises may be used in educational groups designed to reduce or eliminate sexual harassment in healthcare settings. The size of the group may range from 6 to 20 members. The group should be coeducational and multidisciplinary. Every employee in a healthcare setting, including medical doctors and custodians, should be required to participate in an educational group session. A suggested reading list is also included for the facilitator of the educational workshop group.

Sample Case 1

A female nursing supervisor has repeatedly, over the past three weeks, asked a male nurse for a date. Each time, the male nurse has refused to go out with her. The male nurse asks for a letter of recommendation from the nursing supervisor. She agrees to write a letter of recommendation but adds, "I know we are going to have fun on our date Saturday night." The male nurse feels he has been sexually harassed.

Discussion Questions

1. Do you think this is a legitimate case of sexual harassment? Why? Why not?
2. Ask two people in the group to role-play this case. Check to see whether the group members think this is a legitimate case of sexual harassment. Why? Why not?

Sample Case 2

Jack, the director of the Social Work Department at ABC Hospital, has been whistling at and making comments to Susie Red, a social worker in his department. His latest comment to Ms. Red was "Your beautiful round hips add luster to your clothing and make you look like a movie star." Ms. Red usually smiles at Jack when he whistles or makes these comments to her. One week later at ABC Hospital, Jack hires a new social worker, Sally Gold. Jack now whistles and comments on the clothing worn by Ms. Gold. Since Ms. Gold's arrival, Jack has discontinued making comments to Ms. Red. Susie Red is upset and annoyed, and informs him that she is going to file a claim of sexual harassment against him. She states that he created a hostile working environment for her by making sexual comments about her body.

Discussion Questions

1. Do you think Susie Red has a legitimate claim of sexual harassment? Explain.
2. Did Jack create a hostile work environment for Susie Red and Sally Gold? Explain.

Sample Case 3

Each Monday morning, a male physician, Dr. John, comes to the nurses' station and brags about the women he "took to bed" over the weekend. He graphically explains how he made love to these women and brags about how much they enjoyed it.

This behavior has been going on for over a month. The nurses usually laugh and call the physician "Don Juan." When he leaves the nurses' station, they call him "a dirty old man." They say among themselves that they wish Dr. John would stop telling them these vulgar tales, but they continue to listen, because he is a very powerful physician in the hospital and in the community.

One Monday, Dr. John goes through the usual routine of talking about his weekend conquests. A female nursing student informs the doctor that she finds his behavior distasteful and she is going to file a sexual harassment suit against him. Dr. John loudly informs everyone that the student is jealous because he "stood her up" Saturday night. He claims he has been dating the student consistently over the last six months.

Discussion Questions

1. Does the nursing student have a legitimate claim of sexual harassment against the physician?
2. Do the nurses who stood at the nurses' station have a basis for a class action suit based on a sexual harassment claim against the physician?
3. Ask group members to role-play and discuss various aspects of this case.

Sample Case 4

Each morning when Mary, a medical social worker at Catnip Memorial Hospital, arrives at work, Joe, who is a physical therapist, leaves a drawing or painting on her desk. Joe is an artist as well as a physical therapist and he enjoys sharing his artistic works with his friends. Mary complains to her coworkers that Joe's drawings are obscene and offensive to her.

Discussion Questions

1. Is this a case of sexual harassment?
2. Do you need additional information to determine whether this is sexual harassment? If so, what information do you need?
3. You are Mary's supervisor and she complained one time to you about Joe's drawings. Are you liable for not following up on Mary's complaint?

Suggested Answers to Sample Cases

Case 1

This is sexual harassment because the female nurse is in a supervisory role and appears to be giving the male nurse a letter of recommendation in return for a date. This case also points out that males can be victims of sexual harassment by females. This case focuses on quid pro quo sexual harassment, whereby a supervisor abuses authority in an attempt to obtain some type of sexual relationship in exchange for an employment benefit for the worker.

Case 2

Although Jack's behavior toward Susie Red is inappropriate, this may not be sexual harassment because Susie Red did not act as though these comments were offensive or unwelcome. It appears that she became jealous of Jack's attention to Sally Gold and then claimed that she was sexually harassed. By smiling at Jack when he used lewd language, it appears that Susie encouraged Jack's behavior.

If Sally Gold does not welcome Jack's behavior, Jack has created a hostile working environment for her.

Case 3

The nursing student has a claim of the hostile environment type of sexual harassment. The physician has a position of power and authority, and he is openly displaying lewd behavior by the use of offensive language to describe his sexual conquests. The nursing student has expressed to the physician that she does not condone his behavior.

The nurses who stood at the nurses' station did not openly confront Dr. John, because they were afraid of repercussions if they did not appear to enjoy his comments in light of the power and authority he had in the hospital and the community. The nurses can argue that Dr. John created a hostile working environment for them.

Case 4

At first glance, this appears to be a case of hostile environment harassment. Further information will be needed to decide whether this is sexual harassment. The key issue in a hostile environment harassment case is whether or not the environment is unwelcome. We need to know whether Mary ever told Joe she found these drawings obscene and offensive to her.

Suggested Group Exercises

1. Ask all group participants to describe and fully explain the sexual harassment policy in their healthcare settings. Have members critique each participant's presentation and identify those who seem unclear about their employer's sexual harassment policy. Strongly encourage group participants to seek out and obtain this vital information.

2. Ask healthcare administrators in the group to discuss state laws regarding sexual harassment. If they are unaware of this information, strongly recommend that they obtain it.

3. Have group members list the reporting procedures they should initiate if they are sexually harassed in the workplace. After listing these items, have members role-play scenarios depicting how to report claims of sexual harassment.

4. Have group members pretend they have just been sexually harassed. Have each member write a letter to the harasser. In the letter, they should specifically describe what took place, dates of occurrences, and their objection to this behavior. Have members exchange and critique each other's letters.

5. Explore how a labor representative may be of assistance to a union member who is being sexually harassed.

6. Have a group member role-play an employee sending mixed or incongruent signals to harasser.

7. Design scenarios and role-play incidents in which an employer should have known about the sexual harassment taking place but did not intervene to take the appropriate action.

8. Ask male members of the group to create 10 situations they would consider sexual harassment. Ask female members to create 10 situations they consider sexual harassment. Through discussion, allow the males and females to see how they agree or disagree on what is sexual harassment.

9. Ask a group member to role-play an employee seeking promotion and a supervisor who demands sexual favors. Allow members of the group to take turns showing how to respond to this type of quid pro quo harassment and to illustrate the steps they would take to stop this behavior.

10. Allow group members to create a scene in which quid pro quo and hostile environment harassment occur together. After the role-playing exercises, allow members to discuss their reactions and feelings about what occurred in these hypothetical situations.

Conclusion

It is important for every healthcare work environment to have a written policy on sexual harassment. This policy should be available to all employees and should include measures to ensure that every employee understands the policy. In a healthcare environment, employees are faced with the challenge of helping patients with AIDS, cancer, and other diseases and health problems. There is no place for any type of sexual harassment. Sexual harassment leads to diminished productivity, fear, dissension, and negativity in the workplace. All members of the healthcare team must work together and respect each other in order to provide quality care to the consumers of healthcare services and the patients they serve.

CHAPTER 7 REFERENCES

1. Civil Rights Act of 1964, 42 U.S.C.A. 200 et seq.
2. Hood, J., Hardy, B., and Lewis, H. *Workers' Compensation and Employee Protection Laws*, 2nd. ed. (Minnesota West Publishing Co., 1990).
3. Americans With Disabilities Act, 42 U.S.C. 12101-12213 (1988 and Supp. IV 1993).
4. The Rehabilitation Act of 1973, 29 U.S.C. 794 (1988).
5. Ibid.
6. *The Americans With Disabilities Act: Questions and Answers.* (Equal Employment Opportunity Commission and Department of Justice, 1992).
7. *The ADA: Questions and Answers.* (Equal Employment Opportunity Commission and Department of Justice, 1992).
8. Ibid.
9. ADA, 42 USC 12102 (2) (A) (B) (C).
10. *Doherty v. Southern College of Optometry*, 659 F. Supp. 662 (Tenn. 1987).
11. ADA, 42 USC 12111 (9) (A) (B).
12. *The ADA: Questions and Answers.*
13. *Wynne v. Tufts University School of Medicine*, 976 F.2d 794 (1st Cir. 1992).
14. Ibid., 932 F.2d 19, 28 (1st Cir. 1991).
15. *School Board of Nassau County v. Arline*, 480 US 273 (1987).
16. *Doe v. Washington University*, 780 F. Supp. 628 (E.D. Mo. 1991).
17. *The ADA: Questions and Answers.*
18. ADA, 42 USC 12113 (b).
19. Age Discrimination in Employment Act (ADEA), 29 USC 621-634 (1982 and Supp. IV 1993).
20. ADEA at 621(b).
21. ADEA, 29 USC 621, Section 6.05.
22. Ibid., Section 5.17.
23. Ibid., Section 630 (c).

24. ADEA, 29 USC 623 (f) (1) (2) (A) (3).

25. *Buckley v. Hospital Corp. of America*, 758 F.2d 1525 (11th Cir. 1985).

26. *McDonnell Douglas Corp. v. Green*, 411 US 792 (1973).

27. *Williams v. Edward Apffels Coffee Co.*, 792 F.2d 1482 (9th Cir. 1986).

28. Ibid., 1482, 1485.

29. *Houser v. Sears, Roebuck & Co.*, 627 F.2d 756 (5th Cir. 1980).

30. Sedmak, N., and Vidas, C. *Primer on Equal Employment Opportunity*, 6th ed. (Washington, DC: Bureau of National Affairs, Inc., 1994).

31. Ibid.

32. *Bruno v. City of Crown Point*, 950 F.2d 355 (7th Cir. 1991).

33. *Barbano v. Madison County*, 922 F.2d 139 (2nd Cir. 1990).

34. Ibid., 141.

35. *Weeks v. Southern Bell Tel. & Tel. Co.*, 408 F.2d 228 (5th Cir. 1969).

36. *Auto Workers v. Johnson Controls*, 499 US 187 (1991).

37. *Moteles v. University of Pennsylvania*, 730 F.2d 913 (3rd Cir. 1984).

38. *In Re Pan American World Airlines, Inc.*, 905 F.2d 1457 (11th Cir. 1990).

39. *Family and Medical Leave Act*, 29 USC 2601-2654 (1993).

40. Ibid., 2601(b).

41. Ibid., 2601 at 2611 (2) (A).

42. FMLA at 2612 (a) (1) (A-D).

43. Ibid., 2611(11) (A) (B).

44. Ibid., 2613 (a).

45. Ibid., 2612 (e) (1).

46. National Labor Relations Act, 29 USC 151, et seq.

47. *Packard Motor Car Co. v. NLRB*, 330 US 485 (1947).

48. NLRA, 29 USC at 158 (a) (2).

49. *Waterbury Hospital v. N.L.R.B.*, 950 F.2d. 849 (2nd Cir. 1991)

50. Federal Employees Compensation Act (FECA), 5 USCA 8101 et seq.

51. Hood, J., Hardy, B., and Lewis, H. Op. cit.

52. Ibid.

53. *Sentara Leigh Hosp. v. Nichols*, 407 S.E.2d 334 (Va. App. 1991).

54. *Peterson v. W.C.A.B.*, 597 A.2d 1116 (Pa. 1991).

55. 44 A.L.R. 4th 1136 (1986).

56. *Laudenslager v. Loral*, VLW 096-8-196, 10 *Virginia Law Weekly* 1402, Vol. X, No. 50 (May 20, 1996).

57. Ibid., at 1425.

58. *Duldulao v. Saint Mary of Nazareth Hospital Center*, 505 N.E.2d 314 (Ill. 1987).

59. Ibid., 318.

60. *Daymon* v. *Hardin County General Hospital*, 569 N.E.2d 316 (Ill. App. 5 Dist. 1991).

61. Leeson, S., and Johnston, B. *Ending It: Dispute Resolution in America* (Cincinnati, OH: Anderson Publishing Co., 1990).

62. Ibid.

63. H. Warren Knight. "Keep Your Legal Problems Out of Court," *Medical Economics*, 157–8, November 13, 1983, 163, 166.

64. Ibid., 166.

65. Leeson, S., and Johnston, B. Op. cit.

66. EEOC guidelines on sexual harassment, 29 C.F.R. 1604.11(A)(1989).

67. Goodner, E.D., and Kolenich, D.B. "Sexual Harassment: Perspectives From the Past, Present Practice, Policy, and Prevention," *The Journal of Continuing Education in Nursing*, 24, March/April 1993, 57.

68. Childers-Hermann, L. "Awareness of Sexual Harassment: First Step Toward Prevention," *Critical Care Nurse*, February 1993, 101.

69. Zuffoletto, J.M. "Sexual Harassment in the Workplace," *Association of Operating Room Nurses Journal*, 55, February 1992, 614.

70. Margolis, R.E. "Physician's Abuse of Female Hospital Employees May Be Hostile Environment Sexual Harassment," *HealthSpan*, January 1994, 18.

71. Kinard, J.L., et al. "Sexual Harassment in the Hospital Industry: An Empirical Inquiry," *Healthcare Management Review*, Winter 1995.

72. Wolfe, S. "Legally Speaking: If You're Sexually Harassed," *Registered Nurse*, February 1996, 61.

73. McGrath, K. "How Much Do We Really Know About Workplace Sexual Harassment?" *Leadership*, 3, January/February 1994, 6.

74. Gray, P. "Sexual Harassment: Study Says It Comes With the Territory in Nursing Profession," *Hospital and Health Networks*, December 5, 1994, 11.

75. Williams, K.G. "Handling a Complaint of Sexual Harassment," *American Journal of Hospital Pharmacists*, 51, February 1994, 454.

76. Haratani, J.M., et al. "Legal Medicine for Sexual Harassment of Healthcare Workers," *HealthSpan* 10, July/August 1993, 12.

SUGGESTED READING

Collins, D.W. "Can't You Take a Joke? Sexual Harassment In Healthcare," *Revolution: The Journal of Nurse Empowerment*, 3, Fall 1995, 68–74.

Deutschman, A. "Dealing With Sexual Harassment," *Fortune*, 124, November 4, 1991, 145.

Dworkin, T.M. "Harassment in the 1990's," *Business Horizons*, 36, March-April 1993, 53.

Englander, J. "Handling Sexual Harassment in the Workplace," *The CPA Journal*, 62, February 1992, 14.

Eubanks, P. "Preventive Measures Key to Sexual Harassment Policies," *Hospitals*, 65, November 20, 1991, 35.

Fisher, A.B. "Sexual Harassment—What to Do," *Fortune*, 128, August 23, 1993, 84.

Gallop, J. "Sex and Sexism, Feminism and Harassment Policy," *Academe*, 80 September-October 1994, 16–23.

Horsley, J.E. "Don't Tolerate Sexual Harassment at Work," *Registered Nurses*, January 1990, 69–73.

Kornaromy, et al. "Sexual Harassment in Medical Training," *New England Journal of Medicine*, 328, February 4, 1993.

Limback, E.R., and Bland, Z. "An Ounce of Prevention: Sexual Harassment Education," *Business Education Forum*, 49, April 1995, 5–8.

Sumrall, A.C., and Taylor, D. *Sexual Harassment: Women Speak Out* (Freedom, CA: The Crossing Press, 1992).

Thacker, R.A. "Preventing Sexual Harassment in the Workplace," *Training and Development*, 46 (2), 1992, 51–53.

Utley, A. "Survey Finds That Men Suffer Harassment Too," *Times Higher Education Supplement*, 1047:7, November 27, 1992.

Washer, L. "Six Steps to Stopping Harassment," *Working Woman*, June 1992, 51,78.

Weiss, D. "The Principal Ingredients of a Sexual Harassment Policy," *Nation's Business*, 79, December 1991, 31.

Index

169